SCIENCE
AND
SPIRITUALITY

HOW TO TAKE ADVANTAGE OF
THE INVISIBLE LAWS THAT SHAPE OUR LIVES

Dr Brian Gordon

First published by Ultimate World Publishing 2024
Copyright © 2024 Brian Gordon

ISBN

Paperback: 978-1-923255-52-4
Ebook: 978-1-923255-53-1

Cover design: Ultimate World Publishing
Layout and typesetting: Ultimate World Publishing
Editor: Vanessa McKay

Ultimate World Publishing
Diamond Creek,
Victoria Australia 3089
www.writeabook.com.au

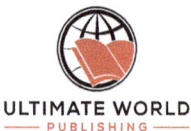

Dedication

This book is dedicated to my beloved wife of 20 years.

The life I have lived is only possible because of you –
my constant cheerleader

Testimonials

In Science and Spirituality, Dr Brian Gordon takes readers on an enlightening journey exploring the intersection of cutting-edge scientific discoveries and timeless spiritual wisdom. This thought-provoking book challenges our existing paradigms and opens our minds to exciting new possibilities for personal transformation.

Dr Gordon makes complex concepts from quantum physics, epigenetics, neuroscience and psychology accessible, weaving them together to reveal profound insights about reality and human potential. He persuasively argues that science and spirituality, far from being at odds, actually enrich and illuminate each other.

What I found most interesting is how the book provides practical tools and techniques for harnessing the power of our thoughts, beliefs, and perceptions to shape our life experiences. The chapters on meditation, self-awareness, and overcoming limiting thought patterns are invaluable for anyone seeking to live with greater purpose and fulfillment.

Science and Spirituality is a must-read for anyone who senses that we are capable of so much more than our current worldview allows. Dr Gordon's work represents a pioneering step forward in integrating the rational and the transcendent - pointing the way to a more expansive future for humanity.

Vanessa McKay
Author and Editor

At one time, science was seen as the ultimate source of knowledge, providing a predictive understanding of the universe. In this thought provoking, highly engaging read, Dr Brian Gordon challenges the notion that science and spirituality exist in isolation in that understanding. A work of complex simplicity, it's a must read for anyone open to the possibility of a world in which science and spirituality together can enrich and empower the lives of individuals, and society as a whole.

Luke van der Beeke
Founder and Managing Director,
The Behaviour Change Collaborative

Adjunct Research Fellow Curtin University (CERIPH)
and Griffith University (Marketing)

Contents

Introduction

God sleeps in the rock
Dreams in the plant
Stirs in the animal
And awakens in man[1]

SCIENCE AND SPIRITUALITY – A false divide?

Maybe one of the earliest and perhaps most damaging schisms to afflict humanity was the historical separation of science and spirituality. That this has limited our understanding of the human mind and the profound benefits to be realised should these two fields of study be reintegrated, is the basic argument and premise of this book.

As you might expect, this is an interdisciplinary journey, linking ideas, theories and science into a unified framework, including practical exercises and techniques. It offers a perspective on human consciousness and its potential to improve, if not transform, our lives. On the way we will explore the intersection of science and spirituality and draw upon a wide range of disciplines, including psychology, biology, quantum physics, epigenetics, and philosophy. We will draw on the principles

---

[1] Ibn al Arabi (a twelfth century mystic)

of systems thinking and explore the science and laws that govern the unseen reality around us.

Those who overcome the difficulties they face and succeed in life don't need to be the smartest, the most intelligent, the most analytical, or even one of the naturally 'beautiful' people, nor do they have to be charismatic. What they do need is an openness to new ideas and a willingness to challenge existing beliefs and assumptions. These are people who haven't built walls of limited expectation around themselves that inhibit their thinking. Success is becoming the person one really wants to be; however, it is only by understanding the underlying patterns and dynamics existent in our own lives that we can create new possibilities and futures for ourselves.

One of the great mysteries of life is the 'hows' and 'whys' of our inner experience; that aspect of being that makes us human — our consciousness. This book emphasises the importance of expanding our awareness and recognising the hidden forces that impact our lives and how, by understanding and harnessing these forces, we can lead happier and more abundant lives. This is a world in which, if we fully used our faculties, we would recognise the remarkable possibilities that are open to us all. Such possibilities can ignite a personal renaissance, creating meaning, joy and fulfilment and helping us to navigate the complexities, bumps and shocks that occasionally come our way.

It's not a short-term fix, but one that calls for long-term commitment and a love of the journey for and of itself; it requires an openness to new ideas and a willingness to challenge existing beliefs and assumptions.

The renowned theoretical physicist, Albert Einstein, regretted the separation of science and philosophy, noting that:

So many people today - and even professional scientists - seem to me like somebody who has seen thousands of trees but has never seen a forest. Knowledge of the historic and philosophical background gives that kind of independence from prejudices of his generation from which most scientists are suffering. This independence created by philosophical insight is - in my opinion - the mark of distinction between a mere artisan or specialist and a real seeker after truth. [Correspondence to Robert Thorton in 1944]

This book advocates for a return to the forest and offers a new perspective on human consciousness and its potential for transforming our lives and the world around us.

CHAPTER 1

Saudade - Nostalgia

The difficulty lies not so much in developing new ideas as in escaping old ones which ramify . . . into every corner of our mind (John Maynard Keynes)

THE ABOVE QUOTE CAPTURES MUCH of the difficulty we face in changing and breaking free from old patterns of thinking and emotion.

A classic example is one of feeling we are simply not good enough. There was an acquaintance that had this belief drummed into her as a child. She simply could not believe her boyfriend thought she was wonderful; instead, she felt he was flattering her to achieve his own ends. This relationship ended, as did her previous ones, because in her mind, she was not good enough.

Our lives can be like that as we journey through time and space. They can be affected by the way we interpret the present through the lens of our experience. The departure point in this book takes me back more than a few years to a time of my life when I lived in Portugal.

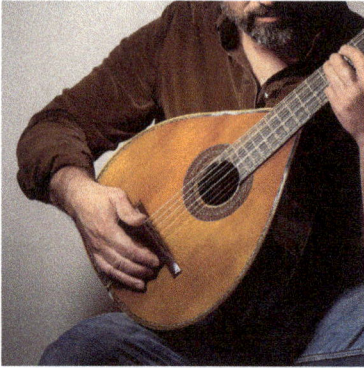

Twenty miles west of Lisbon, there is a stretch of coastline now known as the Portuguese Riviera. As a teenager I lived along that sunny coast with my divorced English mother and my younger brother and sister in what was then a little, undeveloped fishing village, Cascais. In those days, fishermen would haul their catches onto the beach to be sold in the local market. The surrounding countryside, with its mild winters and warm summers, smelled of the ocean and of pine trees. The semi-detached whitewashed cottage in which we lived sat in a quiet, dusty back street which, together with the surrounding activities of village life, gave me a sense of the soul of Portugal. It was there that I fell in love with the national music known as Fado.

Fado music played on an appropriately 'heart-shaped' Portuguese guitar, entranced with its unique, nostalgic sound.

Fado music is the heart of the Portuguese soul. It is arguably the oldest urban folk music in the world. Some say it came as a dance from Africa in the 19th century and was adopted by the poor on the streets of Lisbon. Or perhaps it started at sea as the sad, melodic songs coaxed from the rolling waves by homesick sailors and fishermen.

Whatever its origins its themes have remained constant: destiny, betrayal in love, death and despair. A typical lyric goes: 'Why did you leave me, where did you go? I walk the streets looking at every place we were together, except you're not there.' It's a sad music and a Fado performance is not successful if an audience is not moved to tears.

The essential element of Fado music is 'saudade', a Portuguese word that translates roughly as longing, or nostalgia for unrealised dreams. Fado flowers from this fatalistic world-view. It speaks of an undefined yearning that can't be satisfied.[2]

Ah yes – saudade – nostalgia – who doesn't have nostalgic memories; who doesn't remember the stillness of the moment before the first kiss (or was it the touch) of someone they had fallen in love with? Or perhaps, as you look back at your childhood, it is the smell of a home-baked roast? Perhaps the sound of the ocean while on holiday? Nostalgia can seem a romantic notion. Surely, nostalgia is a harmless emotion.

Indeed, the ability to go back in our minds to times past is there for a good reason. It is there to allow us to remember the unconditional warmth and love of our family and friends and to allow us to draw on that remembrance. It is there to allow us, in the present moment, to mine the experiences, values and beliefs of the past and draw strength and comfort from them.

Therefore, nostalgia at one level is harmless – even beneficial – but when there is such a strength in a nostalgic longing – saudade – that we almost live in the past, what then? What happens when the past takes on an intensity that shapes our present behaviour? A backward-looking life, whether shaped by good or bad experiences, spells trouble, because your thoughts and feelings are the tools that will craft your personal world, both now and in the future. You can't drive forward while continuously looking in your rear-view mirror.

An anagram for nostalgia is *lost again*. Indeed, we can become lost and disconnected from what the future holds for us when nostalgia

---

[2] World Music Central Retrieved 3 June 2007 from http://worldmusiccentral.org/staticpages/index.php/fado

gains a deep grip on us, and we become lost down a line of time. In this form it can become the precursor to severe depression, distorting reality. Nostalgia is a lens that simplifies many of the complexities of the past; it is not a holistic or integrated perception of the times. Nostalgia is a shallow emotion that can deny the necessity for transformative thinking and action in the present.

> **You can't drive forward looking in your rear-view mirror.**
> (Steve Harvey @ IAmSteveHarvey)

Whatever our past, we need to learn how to escape nostalgia's gravitational pull, at least in the space where dark emotions lurk. Failure to do so affects our potential as participants in a greater existence. This being so, let me metaphorically illustrate what happens when nostalgia or past hurts and disappointments govern our lives.

This metaphor involves God. Unfortunately, the one concept in our English language over which wars are fought and communities split is the differing concepts of God. However, in every mainstream 'God-believing' religion on earth, one of the core attributes of God is that God (however understood) is an entity that one way or another touches or even permeates our existence.

For this metaphor, I ask you for a moment to imagine God as creator of the universe, emitting a vast array of musical frequencies, notes, and rhythms of life of which we are the potential receptors if we allow ourselves to tune in.

As babies, we can receive and play back the odd note; as we grow older the notes become riffs[3] and melodies and then, growing into

---

[3] short, often repeated series of notes in pop music or jazz (https://dict.leo.org/forum/view)

adulthood (with all the personal development that is implied), we form a quartet and then an orchestra (although some of us may have more violins and others more drums). We progressively become better able to resonate with the creative emissions of God and the universe in our lives, but then deep nostalgia or past experiences captures us, and we go back in time to when we were just a string quartet or played solo. In so doing, we are reducing our capacity in 'the now' to play God's song for our lives and be the fantastic orchestra we have the potential to be. Yet, when playing in the full resonant and harmonic way that we are designed to play, our health, spiritual, relational, and material prosperity and wellbeing soars.

As an internal condition, nostalgia may be a subtle but insidious obstacle to our reflection of the universe's true harmonic. Another such internal condition lies in the challenges of our past. These challenges may have resulted in a legacy of bitterness, hardship, or poverty or, more frequently, rejection. For many of us this can mean that we are now cautious about opportunities and relationships that lie in the present. We have all heard the expression 'once bitten, twice shy'. As we respond to such sentiments, we tune out of the musical frequencies of life.

Such emotional flotsam from our past becomes our baggage, baggage of wounds, hurts, and outdated beliefs. Its legacy needlessly, and often unconsciously, causes us to drift in a metaphorical Sargasso Sea[4] of our own making, wary of repeating the same mistakes. As a result, we increasingly become non-participants in the construct of our future.

With a bit of self-reflection, we can all recognise how often we allow the baggage of the past, with its pain, rejection, suffering or

---

[4] The Sargasso Sea is famous in mythology for its images of fleets of derelict sailing ships, crewed by bleached white skeletons, and trapped in dense mats of clinging seaweed (http://www.abc.net.au/science/articles/2000/05/11/125857.htm?site=science/greatmomentsinscience)

nostalgic moments, to create chains that hold us to a place, a person or a circumstance long since faded from the present. Such baggage reaches out, down through time and into our present world, eating at our dreams, denying our possibilities, and binding our future with their legacy.

Back in the 1960s Paul Simon, of Simon and Garfunkel, wrote a song *I am a Rock*, which reached the charts in their *Sounds of Silence* album. It expresses the way in which we all can become self-limiting and emotionally insular, as we retreat from past hurts. The singer talks of how he has built strong defenses (a wall, a fortress) to avoid getting hurt. They see friendship and love as sources of pain and choose isolation instead. They find comfort in books and poetry, creating a safe world within their room. However, despite the proclaimed self-sufficiency, there's a hint of past love and a lingering sadness the singer tries to suppress.

Consider though, for a moment, that the world is also filled with successful people who refused to allow the hurts and baggage of their past to impede their future. People like Oprah Winfrey who overcame a childhood of abuse and molestation to become the world's first African American billionaire; or Walt Disney who went bankrupt several times before building his successful entertainment empire. People like Thomas Edison who, when a reporter asked him how it felt to have failed 25,000 times in his effort to create a simple storage battery replied "I don't know why you are calling it a failure. Today I know 25,000 ways not to make a battery".' Notably, Edison also made over 2,000 attempts at creating a light bulb before perfecting it. Other examples might include Helen Keller who became the first deaf and blind person to graduate from college and Franklin Roosevelt who contracted polio as a young man and refused to allow his subsequent paraplegia to have an impact on his life, becoming President of the United States of America. In the process, he became a powerful symbol of an individual's ability to overcome the ravages of one's past.

History is filled with ordinary people, no different to you or me, who refused to allow their past and outward circumstance to dictate their future.

The baggage of our history and culture affects and shapes our beliefs and thinking and so creates paradigms of our reality. These paradigms can keep us closed and unexpectant, blind to the opportunities of life around us. In a brilliant illustration of what happens when we are blinkered, my favourite poet, Elizabeth Barrett-Browning, once wrote:

> 'Earth's crammed with heaven
> And every common bush afire with God:
> But only he, who sees, takes off his shoes,
> The rest sit round it, and pluck blackberries,
> And daub their natural faces unaware[5]

Most of us are blackberry eaters, missing the fire of God (however defined) all around us, with its generative possibilities for a fulfilled life, as we live in our self-limiting sensate world, leaning into the past, unbelieving that life holds more for us. To see the burning bush in our lives we need to believe that it exists. We need to enlarge our paradigms. Such celestial burning bushes only exist on the periphery of our vision.

Paradigms are based in what we hold to be true, what we hold to be possible. They are based in our beliefs. We must create paradigms of reality that are bigger than our experience and more than wishful

---

[5] Browning, E.B. 1856 *The Complete Poetical Works of Elizabeth Barrett Browning* Thomas Crowell and Company New York p134

> **Beliefs form the foundation and bedrock of our being. *Change your beliefs – and you will change your life.***

thinking. We need paradigms that allow us to recognise the unseen universe.

Much is made of the Law of Attraction and its alleged premise that thoughts manifest, or make tangible, a new reality (health, wealth, prosperity, opportunity, etc.). This is casual, if not sloppy, wording. Thoughts do not manifest; rather, beliefs manifest. Beliefs are those things you hold to be true that change how you behave. Thoughts are mental processes. Dominant beliefs manifest, or make tangible, a changed reality. The belief that because you have been hurt once you will be hurt again will preclude you from opportunity. A belief that life was so much better 'way back then' leaves you locked up in a past that can blind you to the present.

But a belief that you can move mountains, shape your destiny, unlock riches, achieve new heights whether creative, spiritual, relational, or temporal, such a belief will change your future and take you into a new dimension. Such a belief, as will be demonstrated, calls down the intervention of forces in your life that are greater than you; forces that are drawn, or are attracted, by your belief as it signals to the universe.

> *'What the mind of man can conceive and believe, it can achieve'*
> (Napoleon Hill – *Think and Grow Rich*).

Belief gives an emotional quality to our thoughts and that emotional quality has much more power for change than our thoughts alone. This is so because such belief will also encourage you to take the steps you know are necessary in your life to realise your dreams.

Beliefs and facts are different. Beliefs are broader than material facts. Beliefs give us confidence where the presenting facts might lead us

Beliefs are those things you hold to be true that change how you behave.

to doubt. It's been said that if you want to attain your dreams, work with ideas, not facts. Dwell upon the result, not the 'hows' of it. Do not worry about the logistics, the people or the money you need to make the result happen but think of the result you dream of. The facts of apparent difficulties and lack of resources will be overcome by the creational storehouse of the universe for reasons that will become clear as we proceed.

Our subsequent actions, which actualise our new life, are the tip of an iceberg, the hidden base of which is formed by our beliefs, and between the two are our values layered with thoughts and emotions. Beliefs form the foundation and bedrock of our being. *Change your beliefs – and you will change your life.*

Do not be afraid to recognise your ability. Move past nostalgia, or saudade, rejection, bitterness and fear and become the destiny that is yours.

CHAPTER 2

Paradigms

If we don't change our direction, we're likely to end up where we're headed.
(Chinese proverb)

Literally, a paradigm is:

1. The thinking that serves as a pattern or model.
2. A set of assumptions, concepts, values, and practices that constitutes a way of viewing reality for the community that shares them, especially in an intellectual discipline.[6]

CHANGING OUR PARADIGMS CAN RESULT from a crisis, a change of circumstance, or a situation that forces us to think outside of the box.

---

[6] The American Heritage® Dictionary of the English Language, Fourth Edition copyright ©2000 by Houghton Mifflin Company. Updated in 2003. Published by Houghton Mifflin Company. All rights reserved.

What does 'thinking outside of the box' really mean?

What is it that stops us seeing and acting on new ideas or even recognising some experiences for what they truly are? The answer is that we have a cognitive blind spot. These blind spots occur because every waking moment we try to make sense of the events in our lives by constructing a reality to explain them. We do this to a greater or lesser degree by looking for causes or reasons for what we experience from our knowledge bank. We do this using the familiar tools and lenses of our lives, so biasing our perception. It's a bit like the way Google's search engine will prioritise results based on a person's past preferences.

Our reality is the interpreted world of our sensory experiences understood through imparted knowledge.

As children this was done for us by others, mainly adults, who came into our world and explained what we were seeing or experiencing. Adults around us drove home to their offspring, their own, often distorted, views of reality, for along with knowledgeable information was some pretty suspect data.

If they told us that Father Christmas was the reason for presents appearing at a certain time of the year, then that is what we understood to be true, along with the tooth fairy's arrival when we lost a tooth. Our knowledge bank contains both understood and interpreted truth, as well as fiction that is understood as truth. Our understanding is only as good as the quality of received wisdom.

When a new idea or experience seems inexplicable in the framework we have developed, we tend to dismiss it, if we even notice it in the first place. Few of us will accept a logical argument unless it resonates with our view of reality. So, such ideas become our blind spots. They exist because our reality is the interpreted world of our sensory experiences understood through imparted knowledge. The interpretation that makes up our framework is subjective, and the lens of that interpretation is called a paradigm. Our blind spots are those bits of life that fall outside of our paradigms.

Paradigms are seldom simply the result of improved logical reasoning or new observations but are a result of a cultural or community perspective that governs our reason. A paradigm loses its luminescence, and its purpose is fulfilled when the context of our lives changes and it faces too many contradictions to remain unchallenged.

At many points throughout this book, we talk about paradigms because they shape the way we relate to the world, to different situations, and to other people. They create our view of the world and tend to be self-reinforcing as we seem to find confirmation of them through our interactions with the world. Paradigms exist in every sphere of life, but unless we each understand our own paradigms, our self-awareness, and therefore our authenticity, will be limited.

Paradigms shape our behaviour because they provide a lens through which we view the world.

The set of assumptions, concepts, values, and practices that constitute our individual way of viewing reality are often not consciously held and so we tend not to challenge them.

If we construct our view of reality through our paradigms it follows that if we change the paradigm, we change our reality. The following true story is a classic tale of a paradigm (reality) changing experience by a naval officer, Frank Koch, which appeared in an issue of *Proceedings*, the magazine of the United States Naval Institute[7].

Two battleships assigned to the training squadron had been at sea on manoeuvres in heavy weather for several days. Koch was serving on the lead battleship and was standing watch on the bridge as night fell. He recounts his experience.

The visibility was extremely poor with patchy fog, so the captain remained on the bridge, keeping an eye on our navigation activities. Shortly after dark, the lookout on the wing of the bridge reported, 'Light, bearing on the starboard bow!'

The captain called out, 'is it steady or moving astern?'

The lookout replied, 'Steady, captain', which meant that we were on a collision course with that source of light.

The captain then called to the signalman, 'Signal that ship: We are on a collision course ... advise you change course 20 degrees.'

Back came the signal from the other ship. 'Advisable for you to change course 20 degrees'. The captain barked, 'Send, I'm a captain ... change course 20 degrees immediately.'

'I'm a seaman second-class,' came the reply. 'You had better change course 20 degrees!'

By this time, the captain was furious. He spat out, 'Send, I am a battleship! Change course 20 degrees.'

Back came the signal from the flashing light ...'I am a lighthouse'.

We changed course.

Because paradigms are based on what we hold to be true, they dictate what we hold to be possible. They reflect our beliefs. How we act on our beliefs can also be shaped by others who might cling to their own

---

[7] Covey, S.R. 1990, *The 7 habits of highly effective people*, The Business Library, Simon and Schuster NY, p33

paradigms, even in the face of reason, and so limit our understanding of reality.

For example:

For centuries, mankind's understanding of astronomy was based on Ptolemaic astronomy, which portrayed a cosmos with the Earth stationary at its centre and the stars, sun, and planets rotating around it. Then along came Copernicus in 1543 who strongly argued that, far from being immobile, the earth and the other planets moved around the sun. This was such an affront to the held paradigm that when Galileo promoted this idea, the Inquisition forced him to recant or be convicted of heresy.

Paradigms reflect our beliefs, and no-one likes having their beliefs challenged, not least the establishment.

In the twentieth century, a major scientific paradigm shift occurred. This paradigm shift is a central tenet or concept explored in this book, encapsulated by the term 'The IDEA'. The paradigm shift in question is the shift of understanding from Newtonian physics to Einstein's physics, also known as quantum physics or quantum mechanics. It is a shift that challenges many of our concepts and, consequently, our beliefs as to how the world operates.

Quantum mechanics was so called as it superseded the theory of Newtonian mechanics. It is more commonly known as quantum physics.

Sir Isaac Newton (1643 – 1727) was one of the most influential scientists of all time and a key figure in the scientific revolution. In Western minds, for the past three hundred years and more, ordinary reality was best described in Newtonian terms. This proposed that *everything is one vast machine or mechanism made up of matter and energy. This machine is entirely deterministic, which means that if you knew the speed and position of every piece of matter in the universe you would know its entire future — just as if you knew the speed and position of the balls on a billiard table, you could calculate where they will all end up. Everything happens (time moves forward) in a three-dimensional space. Consciousness and mind have absolutely no place in this model; they are not on the map'.*[8]

So embedded is this perspective, or paradigm, that it defined the way our Western civilisation viewed reality and, indeed, still does. This is because, in most aspects of our lives, the principles of tangible cause and effect seem to work well enough, even though they might suggest a certain lack of personal control over our destiny.

The impact of this paradigm is felt in all our dimensions of existence, even in our working life. For instance, in this Newtonian world people are a product of their factual details. Perhaps you might have heard employees saying that they were just a small cog in a big wheel. In business and industrial settings management under this paradigm is by control, not guidance and empowerment. In part, this is because there is a belief in the absolute power of logic to explain the world and how things get done.

Anyone who is not shocked by Quantum Theory has not understood it.

Quantum Theory presents a staggeringly different picture of our world. As Niels Bohr, a Nobel Prize winner in physics put it *'Anyone who is not shocked by Quantum Theory has not understood it'.*[9] In Quantum Theory, the world exists in a sea of possibility and probability. Nothing is certain.

[8] EnergyGrid Retrieved 1 February 2008 from http://www.energygrid.com/science/2004/12ap-quantummap.html

[9] Scientific quotes, Retrieved 1 February 2008 from http://xona.com/quotes/scientific.html

At the risk of sounding ridiculous, Newtonian mechanics says that if you throw a rubber ball at a wall it will bounce back. Quantum Theory says that there is a possibility, however remote, that it will go through the wall!

For us to embrace Quantum Theory we have to create paradigms of reality that are bigger than our experience; paradigms that recognise an unseen universe. This is the underpinning principle of The IDEA.

How do we form paradigms?

We construct belief systems based on an incomplete view of the world then surround those cherished systems with high walls to guard against the intrusion of new evidence. In a complex world, forming theories to guide and orient one-self is essential to narrow down the overwhelming task of decision-making. But we face a problem in the fortification we erect around those systems. Dogmas are created, elevated to truths and defended, sometimes to the death as superior to new insights into reality; (Erdmann and Stover, 1993:60).

Paradigms are formed:

- out of other people's recounted experiences;
- from our own experiences; and
- from what we learn of the 'systems' in place around us … arguably these are collective paradigms largely generated by other people who make up our community, culture, or social context.

Without question, other people's recounted experiences are the most impactful on our beliefs. It was other people, whether parents, relations,

> **The undiscerning mind is like the root of a tree - it absorbs equally all that it touches - even the poison that would kill it.**

teachers, or other significant personalities, who explained the world to us, helping us to make sense of our experiences as children. Such early learning, '*is particularly crucial during the first three or four years after birth, affecting the very architecture of our brain and our disposition to think and act, so building lifelong habits of mind.*'[10]

This is now a scientifically demonstrated truth that has been experientially known for centuries. There is a famous old Jesuit saying, '*Give me a child until he is seven, and I will give you the man*'. This reflects an early understanding that the earlier you can influence a child's mind, the stronger the control you have over the formation of that child's character and beliefs (paradigms). The bedrock of our paradigms is formed in the cradle, so to speak. Of course, these other people's paradigms were formed in the same uncritical way. This is unsurprising, as children have relatively undiscerning minds. As the blind monk in the old TV Kung Fu series puts it:

The undiscerning mind is like the root of a tree - it absorbs equally all that it touches - even the poison that would kill it.

So, this intergenerational passage of beliefs and the interpretation of life through resulting paradigms will always provide a limiting basis for our understanding, an understanding that can also be inaccurate.

There is an old anonymous story that explains the process well:

---

[10] The Virtual Village, Reportprepared by the State of South Australia, Department of Education and Children's Services, DECS Publishing, Hindmarsh, 2007, p28.

A group of scientists placed 5 monkeys in a cage and in the middle, a ladder with bananas on the top. Every time a monkey went up the ladder, the scientists soaked the rest of the monkeys with cold water. After a while, every time a monkey went up the ladder, the others beat up the one on the ladder. After some time, no monkey dares to go up the ladder regardless of the temptation. Scientists then decided to substitute one of the monkeys. The first thing this new monkey did was to go up the ladder. Immediately the other monkeys beat him up. After several beatings, the new member learned not to climb the ladder even though it never knew why. After some time, a second monkey was substituted and the same occurred. The first monkey participated in the beating for the second monkey. A third monkey was changed and the same was repeated (beating). The 4th was substituted, and the beating was repeated and finally the 5th monkey was replaced. What was left was a group of 5 monkeys that even though they had never received a cold shower, continued to beat up any monkey who attempted to climb the ladder. If it was possible to ask the monkeys why they would beat up all those who attempted to go up the ladder, I bet you the answer would be.... I don't know - that's how things are done around here.[11]

Our interpretations even of our own experiences are often inaccurate. We try to assess an objective reality through the lens of our subjective experience. This is readily evidenced by the different testimonies witnesses to the same incident will have. Perhaps you might remember the last time you and your partner /colleague/friend had a disagreement over something that happened and each of you saw it differently. It is difficult at times to see another person's point of view.

---

[11] Medical Geek Retrieved 30 August 2009 from http://www.medicalgeek.com/medicaljokes/12701-how-paradigm-formed.html

You may have heard of the term 'active listening'. It is a practice used by counsellors and, if you are lucky, by your closest friends. Active listening requires that you focus your attention on the speaker, suspend judgement on what is being said, and suspend your own way of looking at things (your paradigms) so that you can see things from the other persons point of view; in other words, through the lens of their paradigms. This allows you to 'walk in their shoes', as it were.

William Hatcher illustrated the different realities of our lives as follows:

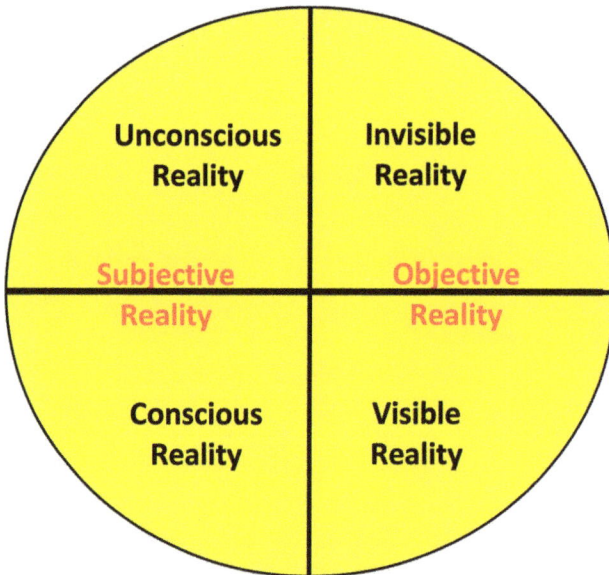

Figure 2.1: The categories of existence[12]

Our memories are the subjective interpretation of events. They are often based on a selection of the 'facts' that conform to our existing paradigms of understanding. In a circular fashion, beliefs are only as

---

[12] Hatcher, W. (1990). *Logic and logos: Essays on science religion, and philosophy.* Oxford: George Ronald Press.

good as our understanding and interpretative recall of conversations, books, experiences, and so on. Yet these beliefs form our paradigms or concept of reality — 'the way it is', whatever the 'it' is we're talking about. These paradigms will shape our behaviour.

This circularity is captured by the authors of the book Fifth Discipline Fieldbook: Strategies and Tools for Building a Learning Organisation, who point out:

> *We live in a world of self-generating beliefs which remain largely untested. We adopt those beliefs because they are based on conclusions, which are inferred from what we observe, plus our past experience.*[13]

This presents us with a challenge as we go about our daily lives, namely that to the extent that our interpretative paradigm is valid or true we can use it to successfully navigate through the challenges and obstacles of life. If it is inaccurate, we may make decisions and choices that will ultimately bring results that are unwanted or unintended.[14]

Beliefs and paradigms are sometimes portrayed as mental traps that block or limit our access to the rest of the universe and what it offers. One sure sign that you are in a mental trap is when you find yourself in a situation you have faced before and can only think of doing what you have done before, despite knowing it will not work.

Respected author and systems thinker, Sir Geoffrey Vickers, has an illuminating observation about mental traps:

---

[13] Senge, Ross, Smith, Roberts, and Kleiner, 1994, *Fifth Discipline Fieldbook: Strategies and Tools for Building a Learning Organization* Doubleday p242.

[14] Hatcher, W. (1990). *Logic and logos: Essays on science religion, and philosophy.* Oxford: George Ronald Press.

'Lobster pots are designed to catch lobsters. A man entering a lobster pot would become suspicious of the narrowing tunnel, he would shrink from the drop at the end; and if he fell in, he would recognise the entrance as a possible exit and climb out again even if he were the shape of a lobster. A trap is a trap only for creatures who cannot solve the problem it sets. Man traps are dangerous only in relation to the limitations of what men can see and value and do . . . We, the trapped, tend to take our own state of mind for granted which is partly why we are trapped.'[15]

To effect a change in our lives we have to change the way we think and interact. We must change our beliefs and paradigms. Essentially, we have to open ourselves to possibility.

Entrepreneurs operate in more open paradigms than do many others. They start businesses in the firm belief that they will succeed where many others would not. Research scientists spend their time chasing down possible new truths where others would think that they were chasing phantoms. Thomas Edison spent four years of his life trying to develop the right filament for the light bulb.

"Before I got through," he recalled, *"I tested no fewer than 6,000 vegetable growths, and ransacked the world for the most suitable filament material.....The electric light has caused me the greatest amount of study and has required the most elaborate experiments. I was never myself discouraged or inclined to be hopeless of success. I cannot say the same for all my associates......Genius is one percent inspiration and ninety-nine percent perspiration."*[16]

---

[15] Vickers, G. (1972). *Freedom in a rocking boat*, London: Penguin Books, p15.

[16] The Franklin Institute: Edison's light bulb Retrieved 24 August 2009 from http://www.fi.edu/learn/sci-tech/edison-lightbulb/edison-lightbulb.php?cts=electricity

Edison had one paradigm; his associates who gave up had another.

Being open to other paradigms helps us identify our own mental traps. Mental traps cause us to perceive reality differently to how it really is but identifying them is never a simple process. By becoming aware of our mental traps, we can change our existing paradigms or beliefs and that leads to an important truth – we *can* change our beliefs.

Once we form a belief, we live our lives through the lens of that belief.

The issue with beliefs is that once we form a belief, we live our lives through the lens of that belief. The problem is that many of our beliefs are self-limiting. We hold on to these beliefs, even in the face of contradictory evidence, perhaps out of doubt, or fear or greed.

As we live in the immediacy of life, there is little consideration of alternative scenarios, of black swan events, those unexpected, dramatic, life changing events that sit outside of our radar.

To illustrate how this can happen, consider one way monkeys are reportedly trapped in some parts of West Africa and Asia. The purpose behind the method adopted is to capture monkeys unharmed and alive for zoos and laboratories around the world. It is also similar to the ways in which some tribes are said to catch monkeys for consumption. How this is done beggars belief but is premised on the monkey's view of reality.

The captors use heavy bottles, with long narrow necks, into which they deposit a handful of sweet-smelling nuts. The bottles are dropped on the jungle floor, and the captors return the next morning to find a monkey trapped next to each bottle.

How is it accomplished? The monkey, attracted by the aromatic scent of the nuts, comes to investigate the bottle and, the nuts, and is trapped. The monkey can't take its hand out of the bottle as long it's holding the nuts, but it is unwilling to open its hand and let them go. The bottle is too heavy to carry away, so the monkey is trapped.[17]

The trap works because of the nature of the trap. It works in two dimensions. One is the sensory reality it presents, and the other is the nature of the monkey's thoughts. One is related to the other.

Because the monkey has evolved to forage, it simply does not occur to it to let go of the nuts and so becomes trapped by its evolutionary paradigm. Like some of us, monkeys tend not to think beyond the immediate moment and what their senses, backed by inadequate paradigms, might tell them.

Consider how many people live on the San Andreas Fault, the largest earthquake fault in North America, or in flood prone, drought or earthquake prone areas? (The United States Geological Survey estimates a 70% chance that one or more quakes of a magnitude 6.7 or larger will occur on the San Andreas Fault before the year 2030). Clearly, it's a calculation of risk versus reward, guided by a belief that it will not happen to me. Like the monkey, my hand is firmly closed on possessing what is in the jar.

More strangely perhaps, is how many people not only refuse to acknowledge a bad decision but continue to implement that bad decision; or how many are driven by greed or fear in their decision making. Share traders know the latter propensity only too well.

---

[17] Butterworth, E. "The universe is calling' Retrieved 1 May 2010 from http://www.inspirationalstories.com/2/233.html

Most share traders will lose money because their hands are caught, metaphorically speaking, in the trap of fear and greed and they won't let go until their losses become substantial or unsustainable. In later chapters on the brain the way our emotional brain overrides our rational brain in these, and other decisions, will be discussed.

But beyond such simplistic examples, like the monkey we can also be caught up by the illusion of the material world and its affluence and may not consider the possibility of a broader, unseen reality. When this happens, our vision/perception is trapped and so our potential is curtailed.

Just like the monkey, we look at life with its problems and opportunities through a limiting set of lenses, an old narrow paradigm. To avoid our monkey trap, we need to recognise it and so become enabled to let go of those ideas that we are attached to when they prevent us being open to greater concepts.

If we are prepared to change our beliefs, the promise is that we will change our lives.

Changing paradigms

Paradigms serve a very useful purpose in our lives. They give us a bounded sense of who we are in the physical world we inhabit and lead us to make assumptions about causality. They provide us with a level of certainty in an uncertain world without which we might go mad. In a Newtonian sense, paradigms define the boundary of what is possible in the real world.

From another perspective, paradigms are sometimes purely artificial, social, and personal constructs or concepts. In the latter instance the boundaries of our constructs, and therefore our paradigms, are somewhat flexible where our constructs of 'what is' brushes up in conversation or through education against someone else's construct.

We need to constantly update our paradigms to better manage the changing circumstances of life. It is also desirable to expand our paradigms to maximise what life has to offer us. The problem is that during our normal lives we do not voluntarily change our paradigms, our core perceptions of reality, very readily.

This is because to do so is not simply an intellectual exercise, but usually involves an intense emotional, and even an existential, struggle. It may feel like having your teeth pulled because you are radically transforming a belief of reality that involves discarding the old one.

It is said that 'crisis brings change' and that is true. People's paradigms are often altered through an extremity of need or circumstance that forces a re-evaluation. It is far less traumatic to be open to change by deliberately placing ourselves in a change environment that influences our thinking and removes cognitive barriers without shattering our lives. For instance, try:

- Living in another culture
- Meeting people from very different backgrounds
- Studying new things in a totally different field
- Trying to identify and challenge your assumptions
- Active listening - look at the world or situation through someone else's eyes.

Doing any, or all, of these things will force us to look at information that falls outside our accepted patterns of understanding; this, in turn, lowers the brain's associative barriers and allows us to establish new paradigms of understanding, opening us up to new possibilities and an increased willingness to take risks and face new horizons in our lives. As William Faulkner said: *You cannot swim for new horizons until you have courage to lose sight of the shore.*

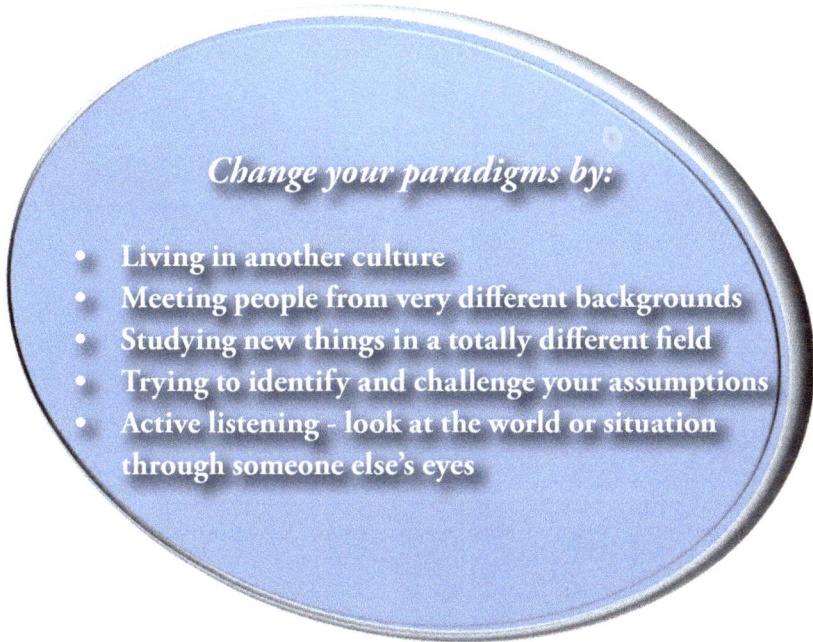

Change your paradigms by:

- Living in another culture
- Meeting people from very different backgrounds
- Studying new things in a totally different field
- Trying to identify and challenge your assumptions
- Active listening - look at the world or situation through someone else's eyes

Figure 2.2: Changing paradigms

CHAPTER 3

About the Nature of Reality

Reality cannot be found except in one single source, because of the interconnection of all things with one another.[18]

THIS IS A DIFFICULT CHAPTER in some ways for both the reader and the author. It looks at the way the Western mind is predisposed to viewing the nature of reality, knowledge and existence. Thinking about the way we interpret our existence is too important an issue to ignore in a book such as this. This is because the lens through which we interpret reality will shape what we understand. We then base our decisions and behaviour on that understanding of reality. For an example of how our lens through which we view reality can change, think about people who are hypnotised and do strange things – their behaviour changes because their understanding of reality has been changed through hypnotic suggestion.

Deep within us there is a need for the creation or the universe to be logical, even as experience reveals that it often seems anything but

---

[18] Gottfried Leibniz, 1670

> **Both Christians and Buddhists agree that the root of man's problems is that consciousness is all fouled up, and that he does not apprehend reality as it truly and really is, and that the moment he looks at something, he begins to interpret it in ways that are prejudiced and predetermined to fit a certain wrong picture of the world.**
> (T. Merton)

logical. In fact, it was seen to be logical for centuries as we derived our scientific laws from its operation, but in the last hundred years we have had our understanding tested as we uncovered quantum physics, black holes, etcetera, which challenge the scientific establishment's long-held Newtonian paradigms or assumptions.

So, what is its reality? How should we define reality and how many realities are there?

For many people, these can seem nonsense questions. Surely reality is the material world that we can touch, see, taste, or hear? Quantum physics, though, demonstrates another reality — a reality that is also based in our consciousness. Our consciousness shapes that reality.

As Professor R.C. Henry of John Hopkins University put it:

A fundamental conclusion of the new physics also acknowledges that the observer creates the reality. As observers, we are personally involved with the creation of our own reality. Physicists are being forced to admit that the universe is a "mental" construction. Pioneering physicist Sir James Jeans wrote: "The stream of knowledge is heading toward a non-mechanical reality; the universe begins to look more like a great thought than like a great machine. Mind no longer appears to be an accidental intruder

*into the realm of matter; we ought rather (to) hail it as the creator
and governor of the realm of matter.*[19]

In the Western 'logical' mind this is hard to understand or come to
grips with because our framework is that of dualism.

Dualism and the Western mind

In the West, with our Latin and Greek philosophical heritage, we
understand a world where certain concepts related to experience are
seen by us as belonging in different categories. Such separated realities
include, for instance, the everyday way we see hot or cold, good or
bad, masculine or feminine, body, soul and spirit, heaven and earth,
or past, present and future. Then there is the way we perceive the
reality of our own being as opposed to that of the so-called objective
world 'out there'. The creation of such discrete/separate realities is
known as dualism.

Dualism can be understood as thinking that the world cannot be
explained, except in terms of two or more different, often opposite,
principles.

We will often see this working out in real life. For instance, as happened
recently, I was complaining about the policies of a particular political
party. Immediately the person I was speaking to presumed I must
support its opponents. Dualism is an either-or position. We must pick
a side and oppose the other. It's hot or cold, good or evil, light or dark,
etcetera. There is no integration between the different realities that
these might represent. Unfortunately, we get attached to the dualistic
view of reality as it pervades Western culture.

---

[19] R. C. Henry, "The Mental Universe"; Nature 436:29, 2005

Dualism can be applied in many other areas of our thinking, such as our mental world versus our physical bodies. A dualist would oppose any theory that identifies the mind with the brain which is conceived as a physical mechanism.[20] To a dualist the mind and body are distinct and separable. Dualism suggests unconnected existential states. So embedded is this way of thinking that it is hard for a Westerner to comprehend an alternative way of looking at things.

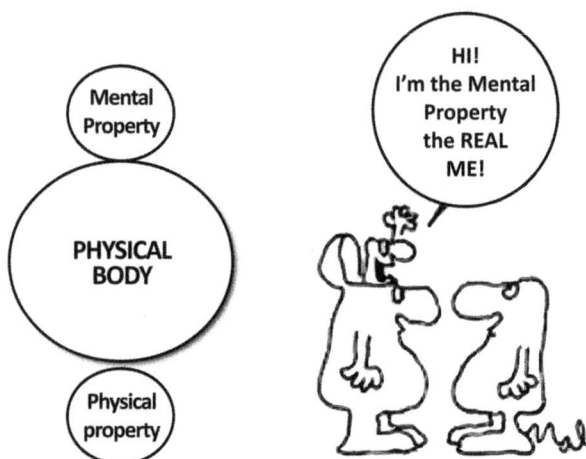

Figure 3.1: Dualism illustrated[21]

In Semitic languages and many Eastern philosophies, there is no perceived separation and, in fact, such a separation between self and the rest of creation, or between mind and body, is an artificial construct with little to recommend itself. These Eastern philosophies would argue for everything in our universe, seen and unseen, to be

[20] Encyclopaedia Britannica, Available at http://www.britannica.com/EBchecked/topic/383566/mind-body-dualism Accessed 27 April 2015

[21] Western Dualism, Available at https://www.google.com.au/search?q=pictures+of+dualism&biw Accessed 28 April 2015

Holding a dualist paradigm presents a cognitive barrier to understanding

expressions or appearances of one essential reality.

When we come to consider the unseen laws of our universe, which are covered in later chapters, and how they affect us, dualism is significant. This is because holding a dualist paradigm presents a cognitive barrier to understanding and accepting our access to the full potential of the unseen in its many expressions. For instance, until recently, the idea of the non-physical mind affecting the physical body was not allowed for in the Western medical dualist paradigm. As a consequence, medicine focussed exclusively on drugs, surgery and material interventions. Now, however, the science exists to show that the mind can accelerate the healing of the body.

How do we change our paradigm in respect to dualism?

One way to open our minds to a paradigm of existence without dualism is to consider the nature of light and darkness. Instead of viewing the two conditions as alternative states of nature, they may be seen as one state reflecting the absence of the other. This is not just semantics.

When we turn the light on in a dark room, the room fills with light, but nothing actually leaves. Darkness does not get replaced with light; it doesn't go away. It just ceases to exist. You cannot turn darkness on.

True darkness, is therefore, the absence of both light and energy. These are not two separate, unconnected states (light and darkness), but rather two *seeming* opposites that transmute one into another. Each is dependent on the other for its existence, for without the contrast of one the other could not be experienced.

Consider the Taoist approach that would suggest that:

All opposites are manifestations of the single Tao, and are therefore not independent from one another, but rather a variation of the same unifying force throughout all of nature.[22]

Or, to put it another way, reality is ultimately a unified whole.

Yet, dualism will seem a reasonable proposition if we look at aspects of the natural world, even the brain and its construction. 'Since the eighteenth century, scientists have debated about the many inherent dualisms woven throughout the human brain and nervous system – the differential functioning of the cerebral hemispheres, the competing demands of the higher (cortical) and lower (limbic) regions, etcetera. Seemingly, our brain systems are dualistic.'[23]

> **Opposites cannot be divided – without darkness we don't understand light; without absence we cannot grasp presence; without evil we cannot understand good.**
> Heraclitus (540 – 460 BC)

Most of us are aware of the left and right hemispheres of the brain and the different attributes given to them suggesting independent, unrelated functions. The reality, however, is that in a healthy person the hemispheric dominance shifts from right to left and back again many times a minute – or the hemispheres may be beautifully synchronised creating a symphony in the brain. For instance, one hemisphere is tracking the logic of what is said while the other is evaluating the emotional meaning.

[22] e-notes.com 'Dualism' Retrieved 14 June 2010 from http://www.enotes.com/topic/Dualism

[23] Larsen, S. 2014, *The Fundamentalist Mind: How Polarized Thinking Imperils Us All* Published Quest Books p62

Similarly, much of life seemingly operates in contrasts. Without the contrast we would miss the significance of much of our experiences. *But contrasts do not argue for different existential states.*

In fact, there are a number of arguments against dualism.

One argument against dualism is the very dependence of all aspects of creation on energy for the interaction of both matter and non-matter (light, brain waves, gravity, etc.). Energy is both the means and the medium for all existence. This is because all created matter in the universe arises out of energy, as we will see in later chapters.

To artificially separate the mind and the body, the internal and the external world, runs contrary to the well-established principle of the conservation of energy and Occam's razor.[24]

Energy is the tie that binds, the medium that permeates, the force that creates all that is.

One reason that dualism is embedded in our thinking is because it has a long history. It stretches way back to the time of the Greek civilization when Plato, who lived 428 – 328 BC, developed the concept of two spheres of existence. These were the transcendental and the physical levels of our existence. The transcendental sphere, by definition, exists outside of nature and creation. It was proposed by Plato that the transcendental is a realm of a greater eternal unchanging reality as against the shifting reality of our experiential, physical world. This is a dualistic perspective.

---

[24] Occam's Razor puts forward the idea that the simplest explanation is usually the right one.

The embedded nature of Plato's thinking in our culture was highlighted by one of the more influential philosophers of the twentieth century, Alfred Whitehead, who famously stated:

The safest general characterisation of the European philosophical tradition is that it consists of a series of footnotes to Plato[25].

I mention this because of the way in which the eternal and the material, or the seen and the unseen, are understood in the Western world.

We know we are, physically speaking, finite creatures, with limited life spans. With short (historically speaking) life spans, we see things separately or discrete from each other, rather than seeing the interconnected whole. Yet, in attributing an independent existence to the fragments of life around us, we create a scientifically demonstrable illusion.

Self-realisation results in a non-dualistic perception – a direct and intimate unity with everything we encounter.

The illusion is that since our senses can readily confirm the many aspects of the material world, then that world is the sum total of the reality of our existence that we should dedicate ourselves to. In our daily lives, in our Western dualistic paradigm, the unseen dimension is a different reality, rather than being inextricably a part of it.

But at different times in our lives, we sense that there must be a better explanation. Faced with our limited exposure to the shards of existence, and recognising our mortality, the eternal question that we individually and collectively have faced down the ages, and sought to answer, is:

---

[25] Whitehead, A.N., 1979 *Process and Reality*, Free Press p. 39.

Is this all there is?

This self-limiting question confronts us when we are faced with major disappointment in our lives, or there is a sense of lack, whether in finances, relationships, or work. We have the idea that 'this is the way 'it is' and that we have to live within the limitations of our lives, hence we tend to stay on the same life path. To move from this small room in our mind we must change our thinking and open up ourselves to new possibilities and to new beliefs about both ourselves and the world we live in.

We need to embrace a more ecological or integrated view of the creation and our part in it.

Quantum Physics, as touched on above and elaborated on later in this book, helps us to understand that our perception is not the limit of reality and opens us to the exploration of answers to the 'how' and the 'why' of life. As we do so, our considerations inevitably will lead us to questions of beliefs and faith systems.

CHAPTER 4

God Stuff

THE ANTARCTICA IS BECOMING INCREASINGLY popular as a cruising destination. From the deck of our ship we gaze at the pristine, white icebergs as we sail past – many of them vast mountains of ice, yet there is far more to what we see than just 'the tip of the iceberg'. In fact, 90% of each iceberg is underwater and invisible to our eyes. Similarly, like icebergs, as Quantum Physics also demonstrates, there is an unsuspected and subtle reality that we could only guess at in the normal course of our lives, yet at some level of being we know it exists.

Since the dawn of time Homo sapiens has held an incurable conviction about the existence of something greater, something beyond the visible. From the early sky gods of many tribal or early societies, to the monotheist faiths that exist and have existed for millennia, we have sought to explain the enigmas of life's journey through our conviction that we spring from a hidden essence in the universe, usually defined as God. Intuitively, we try to weave a coherent, integrated story of creation and our part, however small, in it.

Challenging our ability to understand the big picture is the existence of the twin strands of our universe - the seen and unseen spheres of existence.

It is not until we embrace both spheres fully that we can become more than we could imagine; for humanity holds a unique position in this world of ours. We consciously straddle both these dimensions of creation, unlike any other creature, and so, in embracing and integrating these dimensions in our lives we can become alchemists[26] of our reality, but we need to integrate both into our daily existence.

To do this means that we must believe or accept that there is an unseen reality.

Whatever faith system we come from, whatever faith system ever existed, there is a universal recognition of a 'psychic something' about us that is more than simply our body which is our touchstone in the physical.

> **We can only say we truly believe something to be true when we act on our belief**

Yet a belief in the unseen dimensions of existence is not an unreasoned or unreasonable belief. There is evidence all around us of the unseen and its daily impact on our lives. Knowledge is involved and when we step into what we believe to be true, even when unseen, it should be on the basis of a reasoned trust that impels us forward, not our incredulity.

So, we move forward on the basis of both our intellect and volition. Believing something to be true, we then choose to act on our belief.

---

[26] Alchemy originally concerned itself with the transformation of base metals into gold, but is also a metaphor for how we can transform our lives from the base to the exalted.

We can really only say we truly believe something to be true when we act on it. That is the proof of that pudding.

The impact of what we hold to be true can be summarised in two columns as follows:

TRUTH	leads to	TRUST
Conviction	leads to	Conduct
Belief	leads to	Action

Our beliefs do lead to action and, in doing so, beliefs release the energy that transforms our lives.

One of the most impactful paradigms, or set of held beliefs, that each one of us holds is the paradigm on the nature of our reality. Beliefs are *our* version of reality based on *our* experiences; what we have been taught and what we come to understand. The question, then, is

Do we believe that reality is confined to
what we can taste, touch, hear, see or smell?

How we perceive reality will not only direct our responses to life's circumstances but also change the very direction of our lives.

Our beliefs do lead to action and, in doing so, beliefs release energy.

The premise behind The IDEA in this book is the reality of the forces existing in the unseen part of creation. It rests on an understanding that there is a creator together with a creation in its seen and unseen dimensions, and then there is humanity.

In recent centuries, not only has the idea of a 'creator God' been challenged, but the unseen nature of creation has been less accepted even where there is an intuitive understanding of its reality. In our Western dualist paradigm, the scientific rationalist approach led to the development of the 'technological human' whose right it is to control nature and the environment.

With such a Newtonian perspective which saw a great mechanistic universe the creation was no longer a mystery, but a puzzle of cause and effect to be worked out and God became the great Clockmaker whose universe operated like clockwork.[27]

The assumption was, and in part still is, that the planet belongs to us to exploit as we choose, but it doesn't; we share it. Unfortunately, in the past 150 years, mankind has become functionally separated from the environment as the knower is separated from the known. We are the subject and the world out there has become the object. Therefore, the natural world's intrinsic value to us as mankind has become all that matters. Any sense of imminent[28] purpose in the creation was lost.

The Newtonian perspective has resulted in an ongoing tension in much of the Western world – a tension between faith and reason, between so called 'hard scientific facts' and the 'induced 'facts' that Quantum Physics, Systems Theory, and their ilk suggest (and can demonstrate, as will be outlined.)

This was not always the case. From ancient times until at least the thirteenth century, there was no such tension. Rather, at the time of such people as Thomas Aquinas, there was a sense of fusion between God, nature (creation) and mankind. The creation, with its seen and

---

[27] Carr, N., *The Shallows,* Atlantic Books, 2010 p50

[28] That is to say purpose as a quality spread throughout reality.

unseen aspects, was part of a fabric of existence that supported, and was seen to be intrinsic to, mankind's well-being. With the rise of scientific rationalism in the seventeenth century, however, there arose, in parallel, a sense of our separateness from the natural world around us.

In the Western world, there remains a sense of separation between our so-called spiritual lives and our 'being life'. The less tangible areas of our existence might be seen to have their place but are viewed as significantly less relevant to our daily lives.

It was in a reaction to the objectification of our external world that several philosophical pioneers, like Goethe, Hegel, Bergson, Toynbee and Jung, sought to draw the facets of our broader existence, including nature, into an integrated whole. Despite the following such people as these developed, there was a groundswell of academic resistance to: "the task of discerning great overarching patterns" these philosophers and thinkers proposed.[29]

Many people in different scientific disciplines and walks of life can sense that we are entering a period of rapid transformation; a transformation that is unparalleled in human history, a transformation forced on mankind as we face the rise of China, economic uncertainty, increasingly polarised societies, and climate change with its companions - water scarcity, changing geography and social upheaval.

During the maelstrom of change, mankind has always sought the deeper meaning of life. Throughout the world there is an emergent understanding that the earth is not simply ours to plunder, but that we are an integral part of the creation from which we may have thought ourselves separate. What damages any one aspect of the

---

[29] Tarnas, R.1993 *The Passion of the Western Mind,* Ballantine Books, New York. P383

planet is now recognised to carry implications for all of us and for future generations.

At some level of our thinking or emotion, most of us will recognise the existence of a spiritual dimension, another level of existence, call it what you will. We might not be clear as to what that implies, but the mere fact that we are reflecting on the possibilities in life that reach beyond the sensory dimensions of physical experiences demonstrates that, individually, we are open to the unseen dimensions of the cosmos.

What we understand of the unseen dimension to our existence will, however, be different for each of us. Most of humanity acknowledges, as a starting point, that our lives are formed of spirit-infused flesh – or as Apryl Jensen once put it, 'we are made of God stuff', and this is how we maintain connection with the unseen around us. From there it gets more complicated.

Creator versus Creation

For instance, one fundamental issue we face in raising any consideration of the existence of a supreme being - God - is the inequities humanity faces in life. Have you ever asked yourself:

- How come they got so lucky? They already have everything.
- Why do healings occur with this person and not that person?
- Why do prayers go unanswered so often and seemingly gain a miraculous response at other times?
- Why does a good intelligent person with a bright and positive outlook fail in a particular situation when an individual of great ordinariness carries the day?

To partially answer these questions, we need to consider the nature of being (the ontology) of the unseen worlds. We need to separate in our understanding the roles and functions of the Creator from that of the creation, our understanding of God from our understanding of the universe (the creation) that exists around us. We need to do this even though there is integration between them. When we do this, many of the confusions and contradictions of our existence are more easily resolved.

The Creator, by the definition of the word, is self-existent and 'its' existence is non-contingent on any other factor. By contrast, the existence of the 'creation', as the word 'creation' implies, is contingent on the Creator.

I am not writing to tell you what your attitudinal address towards the Creator should be. In fact, I am not going to dwell on the nature of the Creator, even as we may choose to acknowledge and recognise that we have a divine dimension. Rather, I want to help us understand what our individual attitudinal address towards 'the creation' should be, with respect to the unseen Laws of creation, or Laws of the universe, to open up our paradigms to the possible and so change our lives.

It is widely acknowledged that we are each composed of body, soul, and spirit, yet we are one. It is more than that though – we, meaning mankind, also collectively comprise an integrated and interconnected whole, although that whole is made up of individuals. In Quantum Physics terms, we will discover that we live in a participatory universe where the whole has properties that do not exist in the various individual parts (not least ourselves as individuals). We are more than the sum of the parts.

A truth is that, as spiritual beings, we are not powerless robots in the universe but carry aspects of the Creator within us; even though not I, nor anyone, can hope to have more than a glimmer of understanding of the nature of the Creator. Such aspects give us entry into the unseen worlds of our universe. What blinds us from realising the consequential outcomes of linking to the unseen are our cherished paradigms, or ways of looking at life, in other words our beliefs, surely one of the most value laden words of the English language.

Social, spiritual, marital, academic, recreational, scientific and financial paradigms exist for each of us. Nearly every part of our life is shaped by a host of core beliefs that define our own personal reality and guide our approach to future opportunities and interactions. This is in many ways good... because it keeps us safe, informed and on track in many parts of our life where consistency is important. There are however ways in which our paradigms can limit our growth, success, fulfillment or advancement. Consider that most established paradigms represent the dominant thinking about a topic and as such, are seldom questioned. These belief systems are passed from parent to child, teacher to student or colleague to mentee almost without question. As such, they often appear as an expression of "how we do things here.". This condition of being limited by our beliefs is often referred to as paradigm paralysis and is classically described as a reluctance to abandon our comfortably familiar and well known paradigms for the less comfortable and very uncertain world of the "new" paradigm.[30]

So powerful and durable are our beliefs that they are like the default setting on the computer that is our subconscious.

---

[30] Richard M. DeBowes, DVM, MS, DACVS, *Paradigm Power: How Our Beliefs Enhance or Limit Our Thinking in Practice,* World Small Animal Veterinary Association World Congress Proceedings, 2013

The Laws of the unseen

> **The unseen Laws are dispassionate, unthinking, and universal. They have no regard for one person over another.**

The creation operates in a regulated environment. There are natural laws that govern our existence and impact our lives. Significantly, such natural laws of creation are impersonal. They do not care who you are. Such laws include the Law of Gravity, those Laws applying to electromagnetics, the Law of Attraction, the Law governing the speed of light, the Tuning Fork Principle and the Law of Cause and Effect, amongst many others.

The forces in the unseen worlds of creation are governed by these laws and they powerfully impact our daily lives, hence they sometimes become personalised. In other words, the effects they cause are attributed to the Creator and, therefore, our relationship to the Creator. These forces are, however, there to govern and enhance our existence in the material world and, importantly, we need to recognise that they are dispassionate, unthinking, and universal. They have no regard for one person over another. They simply respond to the frequencies of our thinking, as evidenced and demonstrated in this book.

What is worth noting is how mankind is so predisposed to personalising the impersonal. We do this all the time.

By way of illustration, in Japan, research has found that owners tend to imbue robots with human qualities they do not have. In the Western world, we often do this with our pets. When we do this, it is called anthropomorphism, or the projection of human qualities onto non-human objects.

These unseen forces in creation respond, however impartially, to our emotive thinking, our actions and sentiments, hence we can anthropomorphise their effect on us and give these forces a spiritual personality, for better or worse. There is then a tendency for individuals to want to appease them as lesser gods or look for ways to 'get them onside'.

There is immense futility in this approach. The Creator and the creation are different. The nature of the difference needs to be understood. In terms of creation, the seen and the unseen worlds are different. The unseen worlds respond to our nature within the context of their governing law. As such, we are responsible for that response, not the governing law that we invoked by our actions. If we jump out of an aircraft without a parachute the Law of Gravity does not act to save us, we are wholly responsible for the outcome.

Our science recognises the powerful impact of the laws governing the seen and unseen universe. Yet, if mankind, notably western mankind, believes it will find resolution to the looming crises facing the world solely in material technology that belief is now under challenge. The circumstances in our world are forcing us to let go of the mental framework that is both reductionist and material in nature, for that framework is the bait in our monkey trap (refer previous chapter).

Instead, there is an imperative, like never before, to look beyond to the unseen realms, and to the unity that pervades creation, to find the answers. In doing so we also need to recognise that beyond creation there is a Creator.

What is true for mankind is true for each of us individually. Consider this; it is said that we are created in the image of God (Creator). If this is so then it means that we ourselves are born to create, but the way we can hold on to self-limiting beliefs will lock us into a self-limiting future in which we are hog tied. We need to change our beliefs, our paradigms in respect to the creation, if we are to move on and realise our potential.

Our response to the Creator is a matter for a different discussion to that contained in this book.

CHAPTER 5

Changing our Thinking will Change our Lives

Mind power is the second strongest power next to the spirit. The thoughts that pass through your mind are responsible for everything that happens in your life. Your predominant thoughts influence your behaviour and attitude and control your actions and reactions. As your thoughts are, so is your life.[31]

IT IS NOT ONLY THE leopard that struggles to change its spots; we humans can struggle to change our thinking. The thoughts that pass through our minds are responsible for everything that happens in our life, yet the difficulty attached to changing our thinking should not be underestimated for, as has been said, our thinking arises out of our beliefs and paradigms.

---

[31] Mind Power – the power of thoughts, Retrieved 21 February 2008 from http://www.successconsciousness.com/index_000086.htm

Beliefs shape action. We face a choice every day. That choice is the choice between what we believe we know and an unknown 'greater' truth, which is to be discovered by changing our thinking, our paradigms.

Our thoughts arise out of our beliefs and paradigms

The most powerful obstacle to achieving our potential is our understanding of ourselves in the context of the created world around us.

There is a very true saying: *Perception is reality*, meaning how we perceive things shapes how we see the world regardless of the truth.

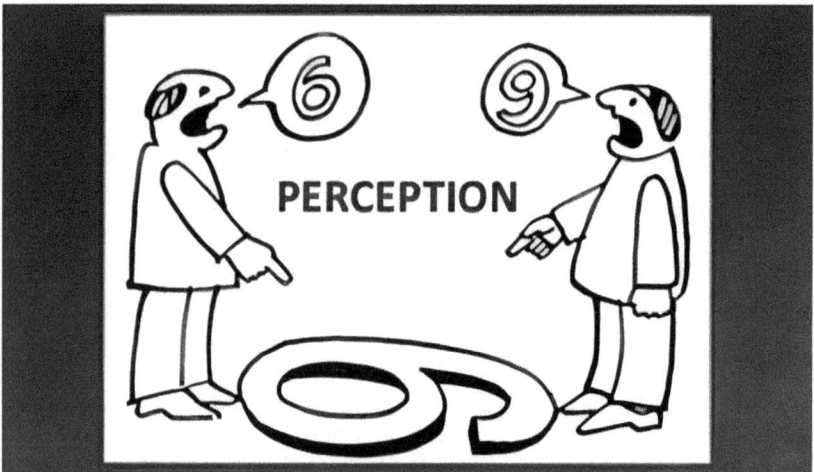

Figure 5.1: Perception

Did you ever watch the film The Matrix? It is simply premised on the idea that everything we accept as evidence of reality could well be false. The story line is that what the heroes think is their everyday life is in fact a simulation generated by an all-powerful computer. The story centres on the person of Neo, who learns the truth and frees humanity from its dream world.

Similar in manner to that film, changed thinking produces a tear in the matrix of our current reality and frees us from artificial constraints on our lives.

Einstein noted that *'It is theory which determines what we observe.'.* The reason is that theory is what we believe to be true. Therefore, we see only what we wish to see – what fits with our beliefs and, similarly, we hear only what we wish to hear.

We select the things we want to pay attention to.

> **We select the things we want to pay attention to.**

It takes great determination to let information that is contrary to what we already believe into our reality. At stake is whether we are so comfortable with our assumptions in life (the theory) that we do not want to experience a larger reality and so our vision is limited. As in the film The Matrix, we may simply not want to be unplugged and face the challenges of the unknown.

The IDEA outlined in this book, like the film, is about freeing the mind. It can only show you the door - you're the one that must walk through it.

How to change your thinking

"The Universe is not punishing you or blessing you. The Universe is responding to the vibrational attitude that you are emitting. The more joyful you are, the more well-being flows to you."
~ Abraham-Hicks

Unconsciously, we react to life's presenting circumstances through the lens of our emotions, rather than responding through the lens of conscious understanding of the underlying causes. The reason we struggle to make the changes we want in our lives, and fail to get out of our ruts, is that we are not thinking about the right things in the right way.

Our thinking processes may be warped.

This can occur in many ways and may be recognised in some of the following tendencies:

- A predisposition to blaming others.
- Personalising - that is assuming that what the person is saying or doing is aimed at 'me'. Sometimes this is extended to a feeling that *'life itself is out to get me!'*
- Black and white thinking or being legalistic - this leads to an inability to compromise or consider extenuating circumstances. We are rigid and doctrinaire, instead of pragmatic and reasonable. The corollary of this is holding fixed paradigms. This thought pattern, which the American Psychological Association also calls dichotomous or polarised thinking, is considered a cognitive distortion because it keeps us from seeing the world as it often is - complex, nuanced, and full of all the shades in between.
- Mind reading - that is we somehow divine how people are feeling or thinking without them telling us. We then react according to our belief.

It's not that we may not be correct in our warped thought processes on some occasions; remember, just because you are paranoid doesn't mean they are not out to get you. These emotive thinking processes are, however, the lens through which our mind's eye sees our world and they will affect our interpretation of reality and so our response, or behaviour.

When we become aware of how perception changes reality, we might become conscious of such subtle cues as body language. We will then consciously try to influence other people through how we dress, talk, and behave, especially when dating.

When we go for a job interview, we match the interviewer's handshake, smile and look them in the eye and we might lean forward to feign interest and so on. In so doing, we create a reality of who we want to be, as seen by the other person.

As Charles Horton Cooley, an American sociologist at the start of the 20th century, said: *I am not who you think I am; I am not who I think I am; I am who I think you think I am.*

So, if our beliefs and thinking and, therefore, our behaviour, creates our reality, then changing our thoughts and our behaviour can open a new reality and new possibilities. If our perception of what constitutes reality is flawed or incomplete (as it often will be), then our subsequent actions will also be flawed.

To change our thinking, we must become conscious of what we are thinking. A lack of awareness, small paradigms, and limited perception are why we make mistakes and live lives that do not reflect our potential; however, when our thinking changes, so does our interpretation of reality.

For example, if we constantly perceive people (our partner, boss, teacher, parent, sibling) as always being against us, we will most likely react in a defensive, combative, negatively reactive, even a victim-like way. If, because of previous negative experiences, we misperceive a person / situation, this too can also cause us to miss out on some of the fantastic things life has to offer, such as promotions at work or romantic relationships.

The IDEA flows out of a central premise about each of us and our ability. That premise is that *consciousness*[32] *actualises potential.* To put it another way, we tend to move in the direction of our dominant thoughts and the creative power of our dominant thoughts changes and overcomes our environment. So, to be an 'over-comer' in life we need to know what we are thinking.

How do we do this?

The importance of becoming aware

We need awareness to make conscious choices. Although most people believe they are self-aware, true self-awareness is a rare quality and is important. Why? Simply because it:

- gives us the power to influence outcomes;
- helps us to become better decision-makers; and
- gives us more self-confidence.

Self-awareness helps us take responsibility for past unconscious reactions and so build stronger relationships; it allows us to communicate more effectively. It allows us to understand things from multiple perspectives. It frees us from our assumptions and biases.[33]

---

[32] What is meant by conscious, and consciousness is surprisingly varied and controversial. For the purposes of this book I take it to mean being self-aware, cognitively alert, and attentive of one's inner and outer environment.

[33] Meredith Betz, https://www.betterup.com/blog/what-is-self-awareness

We must have some grasp on what is going on at any moment in time. Change takes place as our awareness grows and with it our paradigms expand.

Following an extensive study, organisational psychologist, researcher, and New York Times bestselling author, Dr. Tasha Eurich, identifies two types of self-awareness: Internal and External.

- Internal self-awareness represents both how clearly we see our own values, passions, aspirations, fitting with our environment, as well as how clearly we see our reactions (including thoughts, feelings, behaviours, strengths, and weaknesses) and their impact on others.
- External self-awareness means understanding how other people view us, in terms of those same factors listed above.[34]

Dr. Eurich summarised this in the following map of internal self-awareness (how well you know yourself), and external self-awareness (how well you understand how others see you):

	Low external self-awareness	High external self-awareness
High internal self-awareness	**INTROSPECTORS** They're clear on who they are but don't challenge their own views or search for blind spots by getting feedback from others. This can harm their relationships and limit their success.	**AWARE** They know who they are, what they want to accomplish, and seek out and value others' opinions. This is where leaders begin to fully realize the true benefits of self-awareness.
Low internal self-awareness	**SEEKERS** They don't yet know who they are, what they stand for, or how their teams see them. As a result, they might feel stuck or frustrated with their performance and relationships.	**PLEASERS** They can be so focused on appearing a certain way to others that they could be overlooking what matters to them. Over time, they tend to make choices that aren't in service of their own success and fulfillment.

Table 5.1: Internal versus external self-awareness

---

[34] What Self-Awareness Really Is (and How to Cultivate It), Dr Tasha Eurich, Harvard Business Review, January 04, 2018

In truth, for many of us, our thoughts form a sort of background noise, and we are scarcely aware even of what we are thinking of, even though our thoughts shape our lives. We may consequently wonder at the beige existence we lead, or the lack of impact we have in our lives. We do not stop to look at most of our thoughts, the estimated 60,000 plus of them a day, that govern our behaviour, speech, and beliefs and so shape our lives.

The way forward is to stop thinking of everything that falls into our head; stop chasing thoughts down their many rabbit holes. We must take control of our thinking, of our thoughts.

As a first step we must look at our thought life as it exists below the surface of our focussed existences. Our subconscious can tell us what lies hidden in our thoughts through the way we react to the events in our lives, to stories we read and to the films we watch.

Ask yourself why you got emotional or angry or identified with a particular character or situation in a film or story. The symptom is the emotion, but what is the underlying cause of that emotion? Our emotional response is based on our beliefs and our thinking. Beliefs, thinking processes and moods are highly embedded, long-lasting and often unconscious, but they can be revealed through our reactions and so we can identify and choose to challenge them and then change them.

Our beliefs can be revealed through our reactions to situations, stories, and events.

Self-awareness is the foundation for high performance, smart choices, and lasting relationships.

Challenge your thinking

The difficulty in becoming self-aware is that many, if not most, people are unreflective in their thinking. Becoming aware is a major step to being reflective. Dr Eurich found that even though most people believe they are self-aware, the sobering truth is that only 10-15% of the people studied fit the criteria. [35]

In the process of becoming self-aware, we challenge what is learned and what we sense to be true. Is our perception correct and how does this affect our lives? This means testing the given wisdom of ourselves and others by looking for assumptions. Is the information on which our thinking is based accurate?

It's interesting that both experience and power can be barriers to self-awareness because of the assumptions formed.

Many people suffer from low self-esteem, which can lead to two diametrically opposite outcomes: Over-achievement and under-achievement. Over-achievers become compulsively driven to succeed and be better than those around them at school, college, or in work, as a way of finding personal reassurance. At one level it would not seem a problem to be an over-achiever, but there is an underlying impact on that person's health, mental, emotional, and social wellbeing. Under-achievers are afraid to take on the challenges of life in school, college, or the workplace, in case they fail. Therefore, they never realise their own potential.

Neither over-achievement nor under-achievement leads to a balanced and happy life and each carry inherent problems. In both instances

---

[35] What Self-Awareness Really Is (and How to Cultivate It), Dr Tasha Eurich, Harvard Business Review, January 04, 2018

there is a need to be aware of our underlying self-image and to look at the assumptions that flow out from that self-image.

> **'Preconceived notions are the locks on the door of wisdom.'**

One of the biggest hurdles faced in challenging our thinking is that we can come to believe that our thinking is fundamentally fine - it's the other person who has the problem or is a little fuzzy. This was summed up by Merry Browne who wrote: 'Preconceived notions are the locks on the door of wisdom.'

If we do not challenge our thinking, then we will lose self-awareness. So, there is a continual need to reassess what we think if our awareness is to be maintained.

Use reasoning

Once challenged, we need to reason through our existing and newfound beliefs/understandings or paradigms. We need to be able to say that what we now think and believe is reasonable. This process develops in us a mental toughness, a mental resilience, that allows us to make changes when faced with new information or changing circumstances, as well as enabling us to resist the blandishments of our emotional responses to life, people and the (social) media.

Consider it this way:

You will have heard the expression of two people having a heated exchange – one that is emotionally charged. By contrast, reasoning is a cool process. It is objective. Emotion is a warm and, sometimes, hot process, as are the feelings it generates inside of us. Our emotions, and appeals to our emotions, influence, persuade and can knock out the reasoning. Awareness and reasoning can objectify the emotionality of the moment and allow us to look 'at it', rather than being 'in it'.

All of us probably over-rate our capacity to stay rational as our nervous system will prioritise survival over making deliberate choices in many situations. Emotions motivate us and they allow us to make quick and dirty decisions in a crisis. The key takeaway is that we simply need to be aware of our emotions and their triggers to avoid them over-riding reason.

Action brings change

We will not manifest or demonstrate results in our lives without first consciously taking action.

Being aware, or conscious, allows us to shape our voluntary actions or behaviour. Our voluntary actions are about power as much as they are about choice. It is only when we are consciously aware that we can truly undertake *informed voluntary* actions that we will change our lives or a situation. Being aware we can respond, rather than simply react.

Our culture and the moods and thoughts of those around us shape our lives because they shape our actions when we are living unaware lives. Think of the impact of social media and its effect on the increasing polarisation of society.

When we are aware, we can rise above our environment, our culture and our existing circumstances. We can then change them and make tangible what we seek and what we seek to become.

Part of us intuitively knows the possibilities for change this can open for us and over the ages fiction writers and story tellers have capitalised on this awareness.

Remember the story of the ugly duckling 'with feathers all stubby and brown' which grew up to become a swan that flew with 'a glide and a whistle and a snowy white back'[36]? It is the sort of story that grabs at our imagination at many levels of our being, even as children. We devour stories of personal transformation, and we believe deep down it is possible for us to become more than those around us can imagine. Musicals like My Fair Lady succeed because we recognise that, like Professor Higgins and Eliza Doolittle in that story, if we change our thinking, we change the person. There is the story of the maid in Manhattan who weds a millionaire; the computer nerd who becomes the billionaire; the wallflower who becomes the life of the party, and so on. This is the stuff of self-help books, of Broadway and Hollywood.

What is going on in our being that makes such stories attractive? Do we identify with the underdog at some level of being and then hang on to their aspirational coat-tails, unconsciously wondering if their story could become ours? Or do we recognise that there is a different reality that could be ours if we change our thinking and that our changed thinking, in turn, becomes the catalyst for change in our lives?

In The Matrix the hero, Neo, was never going to be the same person he had been once his mind was opened to a different reality. It is the same with us. There is no going back once we open our minds. We are forever changed.

---

[36] The ugly duckling song retrieved 23 July 2008 from http://www.springfieldproject.org.uk/print_stories.php?id=25

This is not the same as saying that we can change other people. Change starts with us. I am sure that, like me, you sometimes look at the world around us, people around us, even your partner, and feel as if we would somehow like to change their behaviours – for the better of course! Alas, we cannot, change starts with us. Perhaps we blame those around us for how we are and what has happened in our lives. So, we want to change them, and we would do so because we believe that our lives, as well as theirs, would be enhanced. The reality is that we can't change the thoughts and behaviour of others, but we can change ourselves and our thinking. If we do that, we change our circumstances.

What do we mean by changing ourselves and our thinking? Research scientist, author, lecturer and practicing chiropractor, Dr Joe Dispenza, described change as 'thinking and acting differently in the same circumstances.'[37]

Thinking is a mental awareness response. Therefore, it is the key to changing our life for, as stated in the Bible, 'whatever we think we will become'.[38] This is because our thinking acts as a catalyst for change.

---

[37] Dispenza, J. 2007 *Evolve Your Brain: The Science of Changing Your Mind* Health Communications Inc., Florida
[38] 23 Proverbs v 7.

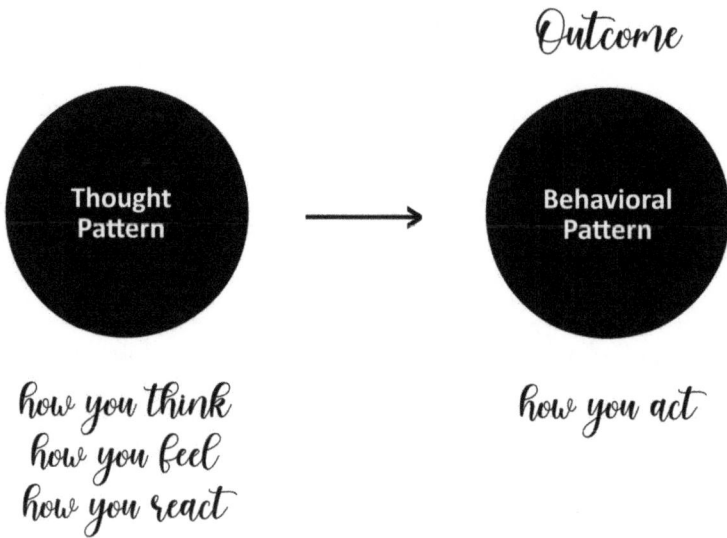

Figure 5.2: Thought pattern versus behavioural pattern.

It is not dissimilar to a science experiment that we used to do when I was a child. I would take some bicarbonate of soda, or sugar, and dissolve it in hot water in a jar. Then, suspending a thread into the liquid, crystals begin to form on the thread. After a day there is quite a community of crystals. It is a bit like that with thoughts. What we think begins to form up on the thread of our lives. The longer we maintain those thoughts, the more they crystallise in the realities of our lives. How this happens will be discussed in the chapter on the brain.

So, when we 'thinkingly' focus our thoughts and then act accordingly, we become greater than our circumstances. You might say to me 'Brian, you just do not know what my situation is like; it's just not that easy.'. Indeed, I do not know your situation, but the good news is that if we are alive and our heart is beating, then we can change our situation and so rise above our presenting circumstances. This is because there is a divine aspect in all of us that gives us the right to design our lives in the way we choose.

The bad news is that working against our divine birthright is our personal history with all its baggage, our culture, and our environment. These factors can work on our brain to trigger responses which will cause us to think in the same old, same old way.

Old habits and patterns of behaviour die hard. This is true whether it's taking a familiar route to a destination, having a glass of wine with dinner or, as in the case of one of my grandchildren, the difficulty faced in leaving their longstanding childhood toy at home. In part, this is because we can find security in routine or what it represents, but habits can render us powerless to access our own creativity, which is why it can take a crisis to create change.

Paradigms are hard to change and yes, life can sometimes seem overwhelming, but we can effect changes to our paradigms and so to our lives and circumstances.

Without strong personal support, it takes strength of character and perseverance to bring about major shifts in our lives and personal fortunes.

By way of an extreme example, I have long had an interest in the rehabilitation of drug-addicted people. In most programs, the vast majority of people relapse into drug use and the best you can do for them is to minimise the harm that they do to themselves and others. There are, however, a couple of initiatives in my home state of Western Australia that really (and unusually) work. The vast majority of those who enter these two programs are still drug free five years later. Interestingly, there are two key factors in the success achieved by both these two totally different initiatives. These factors are:

i) changing the belief system of what is possible; and
ii) changing the social context to which the previously drug-affected person returns. It is fairly said that 'you are who you mix with'.

Normally, what happens around the world is that people coming out of treatment programs, even if they believe change is possible in their lives, relapse as they go back to old friends who retain the old mindset with its self-limiting expectations and life values. In the two programs in question, the change of social context reinforces the newfound belief of what is possible.

In the same way, we too must consciously expand our understanding of what is possible and free ourselves from the way our relationships and cultural setting would cause us to think and act, otherwise they will keep us trapped.

Our thinking affects our bodies

Our lives reflect the wellbeing or unhappiness latent in our thinking. This is because these half-hidden thoughts exert an immense influence on our emotional reality. To influence the way we feel, we must capture and redirect our thinking. But it's not only our feelings that are influenced by our thoughts – as will be shown - so too are the unseen worlds, so creating our experienced reality.

In a study conducted at the Wageningen University in the Netherlands it was demonstrated that *the death rates of optimistic men were 63 percent lower than those of their pouty peers; while for women, optimism reduced the rate by 35 percent.*.[39] It is not that by simply feeling optimistic lives were extended, but that the consequent thinking process led to a chain of causal events extending the optimists' lives. Most notably, and perhaps counter-intuitively, optimists are more self-protective.

---

[39] DeKeukelaere, L., 'Optimism prolongs life', Scientific American, February 2006, retrieved 20 November 2009 from http://www.scientificamerican.com/article.cfm?id=optimism-prolongs-life

So: O*ur thinking influences our reality.*

Some of you will be aware of Mr Masaru Emoto, a creative and visionary Japanese researcher. Mr. Emoto published an important book, *The Message from Water*, based on the findings of his worldwide research. In essence, what he found was that human vibrational energy, thoughts, words, ideas, and music, affect the molecular structure of water, the very same water that comprises over seventy percent of a mature human body and also covers the same amount of our planet.[40]

The significance of Mr Emoto's research is twofold:

Firstly, he found that there are many fascinating differences in the crystalline structures of water when frozen. These differences reflect the many sources of the water. When taken from pristine mountain streams and springs the crystalline patterns form beautiful geometric designs. By contrast, '*polluted and toxic water from industrial and populated areas and stagnated water from water pipes and storage dams show definitively distorted and randomly formed crystalline structures.*'[41] Most of us would expect something like this to be the case. So maybe you are not so surprised.

What is more startling is his second discovery and this discovery ties in with our thought processes.

Mr Emoto's second discovery was that musical vibrations affected the crystalline structure of water positively in terms of their formation when using classical music, or negatively when using heavy metal music. Therefore, he wondered what impact, if any, our thoughts

---

[40] How water structure reflects our consciousness retrieved 20 February 2008 from http://www.life-enthusiast.com/twilight/research_emoto.htm

[41] How water structure reflects our consciousness retrieved 20 February 2008 from http://www.life-enthusiast.com/twilight/research_emoto.htm

would have on the molecular structure of water. With this in mind, he played recorded positive and negative phrases on water overnight, phrases of gratitude, of hate and of love. The water was then frozen and photographed. The water that was in touch with the positive expression of thoughts reflected a perfect crystalline structure. The water that was in touch with negative expressions of thoughts reflected a distorted and damaged structure.

Mr Emoto also tested the impact of periods of prayer or positive thinking on water. The result was the formation of complex lattices of perfectly formed crystalline structure.

Dr. Emoto, through repeatable experiments, demonstrated that human thoughts and emotions can alter the molecular structure of water.

How does this apply to me, you might ask? The answer is twofold:

- firstly, Mr Emoto demonstrated that thoughts have a demonstrable impact on our physical surroundings; and
- secondly, humans are made up of 70% water. Think what our thoughts are doing to us at a molecular level when sustained over a prolonged period and, therefore, what they do to our functioning and wellbeing.

As with our thinking, so with our emotions

Further research has also long established what is intuitively known to all of us, that is that there is a link between our emotions and the patterns of the rhythm of our heart.

In one interesting and quite astounding experiment, research established that:

"During the experience of negative emotions such as anger, frustration, or anxiety, heart rhythms become more erratic and disordered, indicating less synchronisation in the reciprocal action that ensues between the parasympathetic and sympathetic branches of the autonomic nervous system (ANS). In contrast, sustained positive emotions, such as appreciation, love, or compassion, are associated with highly ordered or coherent patterns in the heart rhythms, reflecting greater synchronization between the two branches of the ANS".[42]

This work, published under the title of *Local and Nonlocal Effects of Coherent Heart Frequencies on Conformational Changes of DNA*, went on to demonstrate that not only do our heart rhythms change with the electromagnetic impulses of our emotions, but that these same emotions when projected to nearby DNA changed its shape according to the feelings expressly directed by scientists.

The DNA in question was human placenta DNA (the most pristine form of human DNA). This was placed in a container from which they could measure changes in the DNA. Twenty-eight vials of DNA were given (one each) to 28 trained researchers.

   i)   When the researchers **felt** gratitude, love and appreciation, the DNA responded by relaxing and the strands unwound. The length of the DNA became longer.

  ii)   When the researchers **felt** anger, fear, frustration, or stress, the DNA responded by tightening up. It became shorter and switched off many of the DNA codes. The shutdown of the DNA codes was reversed, and the codes were switched back on again, when feelings of love, joy, gratitude, and appreciation were felt by the researchers.

---

[42] McCraty, R., et al. *Modulation of DNA Conformation by heart focused intention'* Retrieved from http://www.heartmath.org/templates/ihm/section_includes/research/research-intuition/Modulation_of_DNA.pdf 7 August 2009

This experiment was later followed up by testing HIV positive patients and this produced similar results that can be viewed on the HeartMath website. [43]

What is clear is that our thoughts are a creative force, but they are a creative force that can run wild and unharnessed, like an undisciplined child. They are capable of doing as much damage as they can do good. If however, we choose to focus them, they become a creative power for the betterment of our lives.

This being the case, we need to choose our thoughts consciously. Once we realise our minds are a powerful source of creating change, it's important to learn to follow this one simple guideline:

> *Focus on what you really want to achieve in life and not on your anxieties. Your thoughts are the arrows you send into the future. Aim them carefully. Be a conscious creator of that future.*

Engaging the Laws of Nature

As outlined previously, there is a world of difference between the *nature of the Creator* and the *laws of nature* – also known as laws of creation.

Therefore, because the two (the Creator, as opposed to the creation) are different, our attitudinal address, our thinking, and our response towards each should be different.

---

[43] Appreciative Inquiry Commons 2001 *Local and Non-Local Effects of Coherent Heart Frequencies on Conformational Changes of DNA* Retrieved 1 August 2009 from http://appreciativeinquiry.case.edu/practice/organizationDetail.cfm?coid=852&sector=32

Your thoughts are the arrows you send into the future.

Each natural law of creation is evidenced as an observable scientific phenomenon. For example, if you throw a ball into the air and it comes down you can observe the effect of the law of gravity. These natural laws apply to all individuals alike, but you would not imagine that they would apply outside of their governing framework. For example, you are affected by the pull of gravity if you are near a planet, but the further away you are, the less the gravitational field. You will get an electric shock if you touch grounded wires, but not if you are leaning against a telegraph pole. The governing framework, whether understood or not, says that '*in such and such circumstances the law will apply.*'

If we come to understand the way in which a particular law applies to us in each circumstance, we can then use it to our advantage. For instance:

i) We can harness the power latent in electromagnetic fields through the use of lasers, X-ray machines and radio telescopes, even though they are invisible to the naked eye.

ii) We can reduce the propellant mass needed in a space craft by accelerating on gravity-assisted trajectories; and

iii) W can consciously change our lives through the Creational Laws, using some of the concepts outlined in this IDEA.

By contrast, the Creator, as the word suggests, can override such universal laws. The fact that we can confuse the 'unseen world' aspects of the Creator with those of the creation, can lead us to carry the wrong attitudinal address to each, with ineffective outcomes being the consequence in our lives.

Laws are fundamental to our existence. Laws are those rules that govern our lives. There are man-made laws, such as traffic laws, tax laws, and criminal laws, and so on. Society would collapse without such laws.

The laws governing the universe similarly govern our lives, just as they govern the rest of creation. They lend some certainty to the uncertain. For instance, there are the Laws of Genetics that suggests that a vegetable that goes to seed produces another vegetable of the same type. There are Laws of Nature which are the principles governing the natural phenomena of the world. For example, water is always comprised of two atoms of hydrogen and one atom of oxygen. The process is seemingly automatic, set-in purpose and design.

Unseen laws have visible consequences Many of creation's laws, however, are unknown simply because we do not consciously brush up against them.

We may see an effect but do not recognise the underlying cause. As an example, for millennia the reason as to why things fall to the ground was not known until Sir Isaac Newton came up with the Theory of Gravity in 1687 after watching an apple fall from a tree.

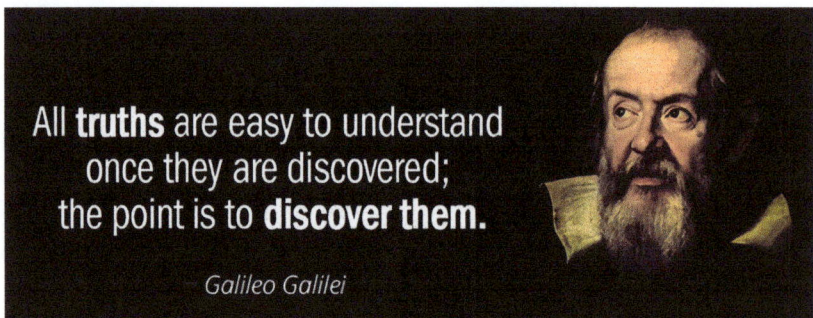

All **truths** are easy to understand once they are discovered; the point is to **discover them.**

Galileo Galilei

Figure 5.3: Galileo's truth[44]

---

[44] https://www.azquotes.com/author/5284-Galileo_Galilei

In truth, we live largely unaware of the laws of the unseen universe that can bring us abundance and joy, as they were intended to do by the Creator. So, to learn of them can change our lives when we consciously choose to take advantage of them.

This is harder to do than it sounds. At the best of times, we are blinded from the unseen by our culture and the immediacy of our senses (touch, taste, sight, hearing, smell). As a result, we can end up believing that some of what we know intuitively to be true, may not be true after all.

Our beliefs and understanding are also influenced as we listen to the (social) media repeat the same cultural message over and over. Remember, the media is in the business of promulgating group opinions, promoting messages that 'everybody' knows to be true. In this way, the media is pervasive as a thought shaper.

For example, consider media messages that imply:

- To be thin makes you attractive.
- Buy more and buy now for happiness - ever heard of retail therapy?
- To look young equates to success - an adage that supports the Botox and plastic surgery industry.
- This political party is good and that one bad - most media are biased in the way they represent a political party and its policies. Complex political issues are often presented in a binary way, with clear heroes and villains, which can obscure the nuances of the debate and make it difficult for viewers to form informed opinions.
- Crime and violence lurk in a street near you - a great emotive driver that supports a 'law and order' agenda, finances security firms, and can isolate neighbourhoods.

- Eating eggs causes high cholesterol.
- 10,000 steps a day is the key to getting healthy.

There are many more examples.

Subtly, our responses to these and other repeated messages shape the way we think and so the way we behave as a response to how we think.

By contrast, we don't readily believe and enact what we can sense in the unseen, even if we do intuitively know it to be true.

- The reason that there are so many seminars of the 'think and grow rich' variety is that we sort of know that there is something in them.
- The reason that we don't seem to subsequently make them work is that we don't believe in the lessons enough to apply them to our lives in an enduring fashion.

At its most basic, we may struggle with the idea of an unseen creational force that would support our well-being. We might then take the next step and deny the possibility of such a thing. It's easier that way. Unfortunately, this diminishes the potential quality of our lives, both directly and indirectly.

In denying the latent influence of the unseen world, we close ourselves off to the possibility of those realms. The consequence is that we live our lives at a low level of consciousness and engagement with the unseen.

This is made worse with the advent of the electronic age. Now our consciousness is further impacted as our sensory input is increased, leaving us more and more oblivious to the unseen forces at work in the world around us.

For instance, our consciousness is diminished when we spend an increasing number of hours in front of the television, game stations and computers and mobiles. In fact, between 2005 and 2009 the time spent has doubled and with the increasing range of online activities that are possible, our online behaviours are becoming more integrated into our offline interactions. In 2021 a report by eMarketer found that we invest on average nearly eight hours a day on digital content. Today, many Westerners own up to four digital devices (television, computer, smartphone (where much of the time is spent), game box consoles and notepads) - and we often use them simultaneously!

Forbes[45] reports that:

> *A whopping 86% of all U.S. consumers <u>are doing something else while watching TV, most of those activities being online or using some sort of alternate multimedia mobile device</u>. But the average number of activities while viewing television changes from each demographic, with Millennials averaging four activities compared to three for Generation Xers, two for Baby Boomers, and one for the over-66 crowd.*

Hence we see the widespread adoption of such activities as social networking through such media as Twitter, Facebook, Instagram, Pinterest, YouTube, RSS feeds, etcetera.[46]

In fact, the internet is superbly designed to take advantage of our brain's plasticity and rewire our mental circuits.

---

[45] Forbes, *The Millennial Trends That Are Killing Cable* April 2015 Available from: http://www.forbes.com/sites/markhughes/2015/03/21/the-millennial-trends-that-are-killing-cable/

[46] Forrester Research 'Consumer Behaviour online: a 2009 deep dive.' retrieved 1 December 2010 from www.forrester.com.

Consequently, the electronic age has led to significant changes in our mental behaviour over the last two or three decades, to quote one eminent scientist and communicator:

> *'we are standing on the brink of a mind makeover more cataclysmic that anything in our history; .... as we learn to appreciate the dynamism and sensitivity of our brain circuitry, the prospect of directly tampering with the very essence of our individuality becomes increasingly likely.'*[47]

Even as long ago as 1969, a researcher, Herbert Krugman, discovered that television, unlike print media, generated information in the brain, but not thought; a discovery, once confirmed, that helped reshape electronic media advertising, reducing the intellectual lives of many to sound bites and slogans.

The internet engages most of our senses with its flashing alerts, the ring tones on our latest smartphones with pop-up advertisements, photos and video clips all demanding our attention if we are stay up to date in our lives and with events of those around us.

This is not to make a value judgement as to whether this a good or bad thing, but to reflect on what it might mean for our awareness, or consciousness. As an example, there are indications we will develop shorter attention spans, living lives that are more instant, lives that are more sensory and less cognitive, or aware. Our lives will become increasingly reactive to the flood of incoming sensations – 'a Yuck or Wow mentality characterised by a premium on momentary

---

[47] Baroness Susan Greenfield, CBE, Director of the Royal Institution of Great Britain, Department of Pharmacology, Oxford University, retrieved 14 June 2008 from http://hsm-science.blogspot.com/2006/05/susan-greenfield-tomorrows-people.html

experience.[48] The result, it is suggested, is that our lives will have less depth.

Such an ongoing deluge of short-term sensory input can distract us from the deeper realities of our existence. For aware or unaware, operating outside of us are the immutable (unchanging) unseen and impartial laws of the universe which govern our existence.

Even when we become aware of the unseen laws, our increasing reliance on information derived through the Internet and social media has led to impaired comprehension and retention. We become 'mere decoders of information', rather than being enabled to make rich mental connections.[49] As a result, the significance of these laws of the universe may escape our understanding.

They form a part of the creation and whether they relate, for instance, to gravity, sunshine, or the rain, they are universally applicable. It doesn't matter whether you acknowledge them or what colour you are, what gender you are, how intelligent you are, or where you live, the Laws are equally applicable in your life. This is just as true for the Law of Attraction, which is fully explained in another chapter.

For now, recognise that the Law of Attraction, like the Law of Gravity, works in our lives whether we consciously apply it or are oblivious to its workings. As an example, if we can feel the feelings of success then we are going to attract experiences of success into our life. If we feel like a failure, then ...guess what? We have created a major impediment to success. As we shall see, this has to do with energy and unseen forces.

---

[48] Baroness Susan Greenfield, CBE, Director of the Royal Institution of Great Britain, Department of Pharmacology, Oxford University, retrieved 14 June 2008 from http://hsm-science.blogspot.com/2006/05/susan-greenfield-tomorrows-people.html

[49] Carr, N., *The Shallows,* Atlantic Books, 2010 p122

Naturally, the Law of Attraction is not the only cause of the effects in our lives. There are many other laws of the universe, some of which will be considered as we go along. Most of us, however, live in ignorance of what is creationally available to us. Imagine if you were given a million-dollar cheque and, having never heard of a cheque before, you simply framed it and hung it on the wall. That is what most of us do with the available creational abundance – it's ours, but it is largely un-banked.

To put it another way, we could have in our possession the most powerful battery in the world, but unless it is connected to something it might as well have no power in it, for all the good it will do us.

> **'Our beliefs are created by choice'.**

The creation, or the universe, is a virtually infinite source of energy which can be given material form through our beliefs, attitudes, feelings, choices, and decisions. In fact, we are doing it all the time, whether consciously or unconsciously. The question is: are you consciously aligning your creative thinking and your attitudes to what you would like to see in your life? Or do you hold self-limiting beliefs that create lesser or even unfortunate experiences for you?

Thoughts and beliefs

What then is a belief that it can so blinker us?

'A belief is assuming something to be true, to be a fact. A belief is not caused, it is created by choice. A belief about a thing's existence is not the same as its existence.'[50] Bruce Di Marsico[51]

---

[50] The Attractor Factor, retrieved 29 February 2008 from http://books.google.com.au/books?id=SqjhlDi73WEC&pg=PA104&lpg=PA104&dq=Bruce+Di+Marsico

[51] Bruce Di Marsico (1942-1945) was a gifted psychotherapist, and human relations consultant. He developed the Option Method. He introduced his method

I really would like to reiterate a most powerful part of that statement, *'Our beliefs are created by choice'*.

What is difficult to really appreciate is that these beliefs, created of our own choosing, in turn create our experiential reality. For example, if I believe that I am a failure, or that no one likes me, then that belief will create a confirmatory reality. I am almost certain to fail or lack friends.

'Your beliefs are the blueprints and building blocks of your reality. Change them and you change your world[52].

This must be one of the key lessons of life:

Perception is reality. Our beliefs define our reality. To put it another way - knowledge and reality are created, not discovered by the mind; or as the popular saying has it: "perception is reality".

Our world abounds with examples of individuals who have risen to prominence through an innate belief about themselves which was stronger than their presenting reality. Michael Jordan, as an example, refused to believe his basketball coach in North Carolina when he told Michael that he was simply not good enough to play basketball. He preferred to believe in his own potential as a basketball player and made it his reality. Bill Gates, of Microsoft fame, had such a strong

---

in New York City in 1970 at a para-professional school for group counseling and therapies called *Group Relations Ongoing Workshops* (GROW). His methods have since become mainstream and are taught to teachers, psychologists, therapists, social workers, clergy and other practitioners as an additional tool in their professions. The foundation of his approach to helping people was based on his recognition that people were unhappy because they believed that they should be, for whatever reason – the choice was theirs.

52 Email 8 May 2008 Enoch Mind Reality

belief in what he was about that he dropped out of college and set up his business in a motel in Albuquerque, New Mexico, next to some prostitutes. The rest is history. The list goes on and on.

It is a universal truth that to affect a change we must attempt a cognitive or deliberate restructuring of thoughts and beliefs. The problem is that our thoughts and beliefs are so ingrained that they form our assumptions about life and it is hard to even recognise them - but recognise them we must.

Our thoughts, assumptions and beliefs are entwined and, because beliefs define our reality, they shape the level to which we achieve our goals. If we subconsciously do not believe in our ability or circumstances to achieve our goals, then we have sabotaged our life's journey before we even start. Therefore, our beliefs, as well as our thoughts, are not just important, they are crucial.

Many of our beliefs are formed in childhood, yet they still affect our lives today - in every moment! The thing to think about is the fact that we have a belief about everything in our world.

Some of these beliefs support us, some limit us. Our beliefs create patterns of behaviour and then these beliefs are confirmed because our behaviour creates a reality which reinforces our paradigms. This is the real 'Catch 22'[53] of life.

Have you ever woken up one day and, tripping over the cat or spilling a cup of coffee, you just know it's going to be a bad day? Lo and behold, what happens? A thousand little things seem to go wrong and so you come home and say 'well, I just knew it was going to be a bad day, I

---

[53] Catch 22 was the term coined by the novelist Joseph Heller in his book by the same name that describes a paradox of cause and effect.

should have stayed in bed.' Think though, who created this day first in your mind and then in your life?

If things keep happening in your life that you really don't desire consciously, it may simply mean that there is a belief at a subconscious level that is undermining you. Maybe it is a belief about a lack of your personal worthiness, ability, or possibility in life. Our beliefs are the building blocks of our reality. They are also the blockers of change. As we saw in the previous chapter, our beliefs shape our paradigms.

Change your beliefs, then you change your paradigms, and you change your reality.

At its most elemental and stunning is the way our beliefs affect our life expectancy. As distinguished author and medical practitioner, Dr Christiane Northrup, wrote:

> *'Think positively. Studies have shown that expecting the worst is linked to a 25 percent higher risk of dying before age 65. If that isn't evidence of a mind-body connection, I don't know what is.'*[54]

Studies have shown that expecting the worst is linked to a 25 percent higher risk of dying before age 65

Everybody's life has certain sticking points. These are events that keep recurring in one form or another until we recognise that we must change our thinking and so our behaviour. How can we identify where those sticking points are?

---

[54] Christiane Northrup MD Retrieved 16 July 2008 from http://www.drnorthrup.com/inspiration/index.php

Ask yourself:

- What is the reality I am currently experiencing? Good relationships, enjoyable work, a fulfilling life ... or ...

- What patterns of events keep re-occurring? Maybe you change jobs, relationships, etcetera., and after the exciting opening moments the old familiar patterns leak into the new. Is this your experience? What are those patterns and why is it they reoccur?

- What sorts of problems keep on arising in my life? Are they in the area of health, wealth, or relationships? Pause for a moment and consider this question.

This book is a philosophical romp into the possible (which I have called the IDEA), simply because the world we live in is to no small degree a reflection of our perception of it. Change our perception, change our lives. At its most basic, life seen as a glass half full will have different outcomes to a life seen as a glass half empty.

This is not a new truth. It is a truth that has been understood by some for centuries. It's the basis for motivational films, books, and seminars and many a self-help program.

How is it we hear significant truths, know them instinctively to be life changing, and then lose sight of them in the hurly-burly of our everyday existence, even though in our own lives we hear stories of people overcoming the odds.

There is poem written by Walter D. Wintle that goes as follows:

If you think you are beaten, you are.
If you think you dare not, you don't.
If you'd like to win but you think you can't,
It's almost certain you won't.

Life's battles don't always go
To the stronger or faster man;
But sooner or later the man who wins,
Is the one who thinks he can.

We hear of ninety-year-olds winning a Salsa competition, of a paraplegic climbing Everest or walking the Kokoda trail, of orphans brought up with staggering disadvantage becoming highly successful business people. They are the over-comers of life's circumstances.

We know these stories as truths, so how is it that we still struggle to lose weight, stay on a diet, secure the job we want, meet that special person, or control our moods? You might then ask: How do I become an over-comer?

The IDEA contains the answer, but there is a difference to knowing something and to applying it effectually in our lives. Once we know the truth, we need to make it our journey to continue to expand both our awareness and our commitment to using that truth. It's not a glamorous journey, but neither is it boring. Was learning to walk glamorous?

Awareness is power because awareness gives you choice.

True learning is about discovering ourselves and how we can create our lives at every level. Awareness is about being conscious of our inner and outer environment. Awareness is power; the more you have it, the more power you have over every area of life. Awareness is power because awareness gives you choice. The vehicle on this journey is our mind.

Universally, in all ages, both in scientific frameworks and faith systems, the ability of the mind to change our lives and our life circumstances is a given.

Why is that? Why is this understanding so universal? The answer is simple – it is a feature of human design. Such a persistent and universal conviction is born out of the experience of the many that have gone before us. They are the many who would encourage us even now to seize the moment and then live a life scarcely conceived. Just consider a very few statements from a very diverse set of people:

'Your unconscious -mind... [has a] power that turns wishes into realities when the wishes are strong enough.' [55]

'Be the change that you want to see in the world.' [56]

'Creation is always happening. Every time an individual has a thought, or a prolonged chronic way of thinking, they are in a creation process. Something is going to manifest out of those thoughts.' [57]

'I tell you the truth if you have faith and do not doubt ..... You can say to this mountain, 'Go throw yourself into the sea,' it will be done.' [58]

---

[55] Norman V. Peale *positive imaging* p.77

[56] Mahatma Gandhi Retrieved 23 July 2007 from http://www.favorite-famous-quotes.com/famous-ghandi-quotes.html

[57] Beckwith, M. B. quoted by Byrne, R. 2006 *The Secret* Simon and Schuster Inc. United States of America p16

[58] 'Mathew 21:21' 1978 *The Holy Bible New International Version* Zondervan Bible Publishers Michigan USA

'At a fundamental level there is no separation between our internal life and our immediate circumstances. Therefore, the causes we make through our thought, word and action manifest in our external surroundings.'[59]

Even in the dry and dusty halls of the Harvard Business School we find the same sentiment. William George, past CEO and Professor of Management Practice at Harvard Business School, stated that *'we are all spiritual beings, composed of minds, bodies, and a spiritual side. To unleash the whole capacity of the individual - mind body and spirit - gives enormous power.'*[60]

If we are to positively change our lives, the thread through it all is a faith or belief in ourselves; a faith that how we think really makes a difference because it not only affects our actions but also because such 'faith' touches the unseen worlds around us. It connects us to a higher plain for: *'faith is the [substance] of things hoped for, the evidence of things not seen.'*[61]

Why is this?

As walking aerials in a participatory universe, we behave as continuously thinking, creating, reflecting beings who act as radio stations. Like any television or radio, we can tune into different frequencies. Hence the Universal Law:

---

[59] Buddhism: Oneness of life and its environment retrieved 23 July 2007 from http://www.sgi-uk.org/index.php/buddhism/oneness

[60] Buddhism: Oneness of life and its environment retrieved 23 July 2007 from http://www.sgi-uk.org/index.php/buddhism/onenessdership.pdf

[61] Hebrews 11:1 1978 *The Holy Bible New International Version* Zondervan Bible Publishers Michigan USA

What you think about shapes your life and what you tune into you get.

Wherever thought goes, a chemical goes with it

All beliefs have accompanying emotions that act as signatures of those beliefs. The stronger the belief, the stronger, more charged, and distinct the emotions will be that surround it. The more charged and distinct the emotions, the more chemicals will flood your body, aligning your body with your mind. As Dr Deepak Chopra writes in Ageless Body, Timeless Mind, *'Without the feeling there is no hormone; without the hormone there is no feeling . . . The revolution we call mind-body medicine was based on this simple discovery: wherever thought goes, a chemical goes with it.'*[62]

In a similar fashion, the way we live our lives carries a signature signal into the universe that is uniquely ours, and that signature reflects our beliefs, values, and attitudes. Each person walking this earth is constantly sending out such signals into the unseen universe, the quantum holder of the life force of our existence. If that signal is less than optimal, then that signature can be changed by you.

Is your signature rock 'n' roll, classical, or the Rocky Horror show?

Along with death and taxes, one great certainty in life is that the unseen universe will strongly respond to our signals.

How many times have you heard a statement similar to: *what you think about you become* or *what you tune into you get?* You, along with many others, may say: I understand this and will now do something about it.

---

[62] The Huffington Post Retrieved 29 September 2008 from http://www.huffingtonpost.com/deb-shapiro/embodymindem-just-one-big_b_128794.html

In reality, however, it is not so simple. Why? This is because:

1. We need to tap into a higher form of life than our material life of external experiences; in fact, it is an aspirational inner life;
2. We need to over-ride and reprint our existing patterns of thinking, enhancing our self-beliefs and so our expectations in life and relationships; and
3. We need to integrate our inner world[63] with its paradigms and our outer world with the unseen. To do this, we have to tune into a higher frequency (if we are to maintain the radio analogy).

Remembering that beliefs shape behaviour and how we think can limit our choices, where do we start in changing our paradigms?

One strategy to help broaden our thinking, among several detailed in this book, and to help begin to reprint our existing patterns of behaviour, is 'systems thinking'.

---

[63] We all have an inner world that is quite distinct from the outer world we encounter with our physical senses. It is the world we meet when we have an emotional reaction, an idea, or close our eyes and live in our fantasies, imagination or dreams http://dreamhawk.com/inner-life/inner-world/

Systems Thinking changes our perception of reality

How do we understand reality, and can we change it?

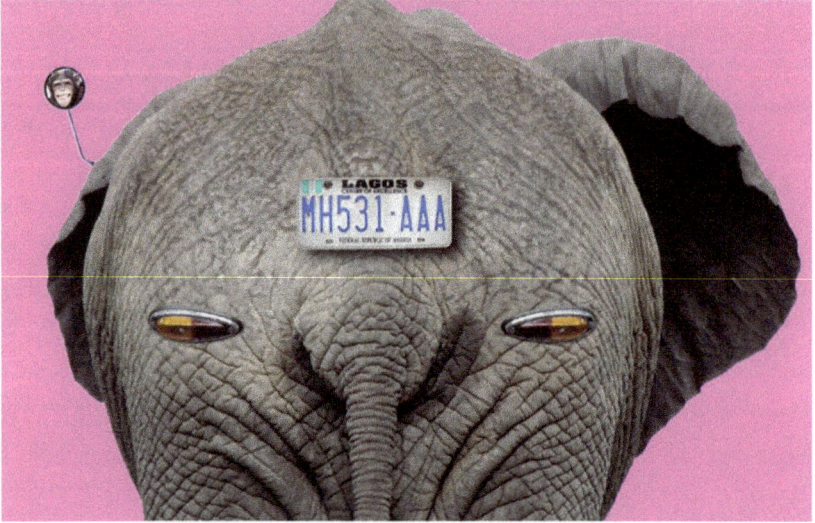

There is an ancient Sufi story of an elephant and some blind men which goes as follows:

Once there was a city, the inhabitants of which were all blind. They had heard of elephants and were curious to see [sic] one face to face. They were still full of this desire when one day a caravan arrived and camped outside the city. There was an elephant in the caravan. When the inhabitants of the city heard there was an elephant in the caravan, the wisest and most intelligent men of the city decided to go out and see the elephant. A number of them left the city and went to the place where the elephant was. One stretched out his hands, grasped the elephant's ear, and perceived something resembling a fan. Another stretched out his hands, grasped the elephant's trunk, and perceived something resembling a snake. This man decided that the elephant looked like a snake. A third stretched out his hands, grasped the elephant's leg, and perceived something like a tree. He decided that the elephant looked like a tree. A fourth stretched his hands, grasped the elephant's tusk, and perceived something like a spear. He decided that the elephant looked like a weapon. Delighted, they all returned to the city. After each one had gone back to his quarter, the people asked: "Did you see the elephant?" Each one answered yes. They asked: "What does he look like? What kind of shape has he?" Then one in his quarter replied: "The elephant looks like a fan. And the second man in the second quarter: "The elephant looks like a snake." The third man in the third quarter: "The elephant looks like a tree." And the fourth man in fourth quarter: "The elephant looks like a weapon." And inhabitants of each quarter formed their opinion in accord; with what they had heard.[64]

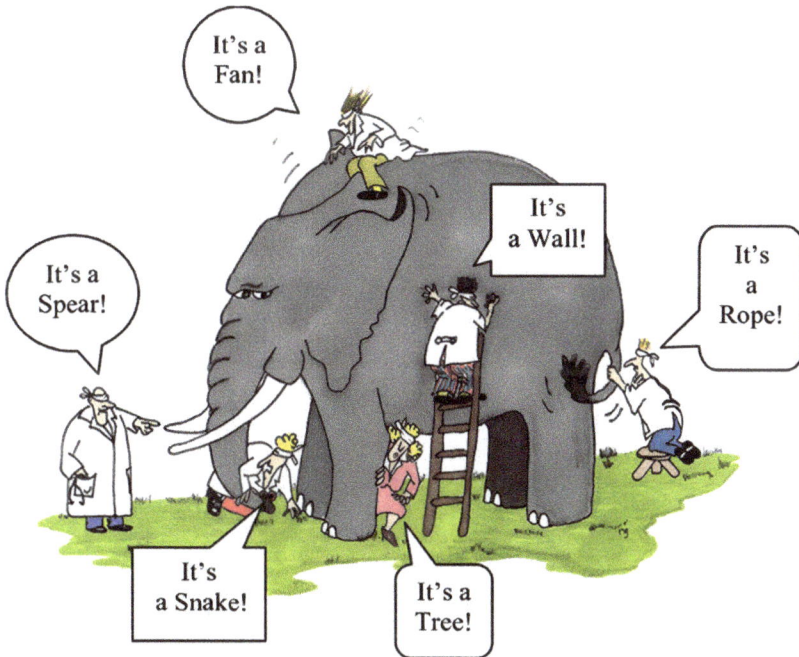

Figure 5.4: The blind people and the elephant

[64] https://sufiway.eu/sufi-story-elephant-blind-men/ accessed 8 June 2022

The blind men and the elephant – everyone sees only a part of a more complex reality and tends to assume that what they see is the whole picture.

It is easy to confuse the part of reality we engage with as the whole. It is easy to confuse the part of reality we engage with as the whole. Everything around us is a system, and every system is part of another system. By understanding how things around us interlink, we become better at seeing how things work together and how these same things can be manipulated, changed, and modified to our advantage. This process is called Systems Thinking.[65]

There is a fundamental mismatch between the nature of reality in complex systems and our predominant ways of thinking about that reality. Structures of which we are unaware hold us prisoner. For instance, our current daily routine is a system (but we often see it linearly). We get up; we brush our teeth; we go to work; we consume information; we do actual work that earns an income; we talk to people, etcetera. If we do these same things for 20 years, we'll probably do the same things for the rest of our life. Our system defines both our present reality and our future reality.

Conversely, learning to see the structures within which we operate begins a process of freeing ourselves from previously unseen forces and, ultimately, mastering the ability to work with them and change them.[66] Being aware allows you to change them and so your future.

---

[65] https://durmonski.com/life-advice/use-systems-thinking-in-daily-life/
[66] The Fifth Discipline: The Art and Practice of the Learning Organization (Century business). Random House.

Don't be put off by the term Systems Thinking – it is simply a way of making sense of the complexity of the world by looking at it in terms of wholes and relationships, rather than by splitting it down into its parts.[67] At its best, Systems Thinking helps us to stop thinking from crisis to crisis and approach the issues we face in a more integrated way.

Systems come in all shapes and sizes. Systems Thinking now pervades many aspects of business, science, and government because it helps us to better understand our problems and identify how to promote positive change. It also offers us insights and can be quite revealing! Systems Thinking is concerned with revealing truths, where the unseen is just as important as the seen. Think of the elephant story.

Linda Sweeney and Dennis Booth, from years of working in this area, defined a systems thinker as someone who:

- Sees the whole picture.
- Changes perspectives, seeing new ways of approaching an issue.
- Looks for interdependencies.
- Considers how mental models (paradigms of how things work) create our future.
- Gives attention to the long term.
- 'Goes wide' to see complex cause and effect relationships.
- Finds where unanticipated consequences emerge.
- Focuses on the structure of the system and not blame.
- Sees oneself as part of and not outside the system.
- Watches out for win / lose mindsets, knowing that they usually make matters worse in situations of high interdependence.[68]

[67] Magnus Ramage and Karen Shipp. 2009. Systems Thinkers. Springer

[68] *The Systems Thinking Playbook: Exercises to Stretch and Build Learning and Systems Thinking Capabilities* Linda Booth Sweeney, Dennis Meadows Chelsea Green Publishing, 2010

One of the components of Systems Thinking is recognition that, *'at different levels, observed phenomena exhibit properties that do not exist at lower levels. They are called emergent properties since they only emerge at that particular level.'* [69]

As an example of an emergent property, think of your favourite team sport, whether cricket or baseball, netball or soccer, rugby, or grid iron. Many of those who follow a team sport would fantasise about the creation of a dream team by identifying spectacular individuals that they would include. This is essentially what team club management does. In reality, however, one cannot always predict the success of a team by looking at individual player performance. It is really about what emerges when these talented individuals come together as a team.

Another example, in our earlier example of water, you could not have predicted the emergent properties of oxygen and hydrogen when they come together and then form this non-gaseous substance that we know as water. Or in chemistry, for example, the taste of saltiness is a property of salt, but that does not mean that it is also a property of sodium or chlorine, the two elements which make up salt. Thus, saltiness is an emergent or a supervenient property of salt.

In our society a common emergent property is distortion of information when errors accumulate as information passes through a social network, such as social media. This emergent property reminds me of the party game of 'telephone', which starts by giving a secret message to one person in a group. That person whispers the message to a second person, and the message is whispered from one person to another. After everyone has been told the message, the first person and last person tell everyone the message as they understood it. To everyone's

---

[69] Capra, F 1996 *The web of life* HarperCollins Publishers London p37

amusement, the last person's version of the message is typically incorrect, even though the last person is not a liar.

> **A failure to realise that a property is emergent can lead us to serious errors of judgement.**

A failure to realise that a property is emergent can lead us to serious errors of judgement; similarly, once aware of emergent properties, it is easier for us to see what is really happening. When something adverse happens, our immediate reaction is often to locate the cause and to apply a fix; however, this 'fix' will have effects of its own, and very often these are not positive ones.

Emergent properties will affect the way we interact at many levels of existence. They sit at the heart of the concept of Systems Thinking as the behaviour of a system is an emergent property of its structure, not of its parts.

As Donella H. Meadows put it:

> *Once we see the relationship between structure and behaviour, we can begin to understand how systems work, what makes them produce poor results, and how to shift them into better behaviour patterns. As our world continues to change rapidly and become more complex, systems thinking will help us manage, adapt, and see the wide range of choices we have before us.*[70]

Significantly, she writes: '*systems can change themselves utterly by creating whole new structures and behaviours.*'

---

[70] Donella H. Meadows, Thinking in Systems, 2008

97

As discussed, in our Newtonian world we have been taught to think linearly using our rational ability to trace direct paths from cause to effect, looking at things in small and understandable pieces; but *'we can complement that way of seeing and thinking with a more intuitive way, a way that allows us to stop casting blame and to see the system as the source of its own problems, and find the courage and wisdom to restructure it.'*[71]

Systems Thinking is concerned with revealing truths of nature, where the unseen is just as important as the seen. As a starting point, we do this through inquiry into the reasons, the foundations, the meanings, and the ways of the unseen. This both broadens our paradigms and allows us to transcend them - changing our beliefs and our attitudinal address to life.

- Systems Thinking allows us to appreciate the non-obvious, as well as the obvious ways we are connected to each other.
- Systems Thinking helps us recognise the unintended impacts of our intentions, thinking, and actions on others, as well as ourselves.
- Systems Thinking helps us apply this self-awareness to changing how we relate to others in our system.

The trick to succeeding in our inquiry is to recognise which of our behaviours result from systems and what conditions release those behaviours. In this way, we can work to rearrange the structures and conditions of the system to reduce the likelihood of self-destructive behaviours, such as addiction, and encourage more positive behaviours.

This requires self-awareness. To build self-awareness, we must try to sense our own boundaries and limitations. By being clear about

---

[71] Adriano Machado, Embrace your Journey #22, 5 June 2022

ourselves and our abilities, gifts, and limitations, we can see the larger system much more clearly.

Succeeding chapters in this book outline aspects of such an inquiry and demonstrate the science behind the thinking.

Because the philosophy outlined in The IDEA contained in this book is not based on wishful thinking but is a pointer about the way things have always been in time and space, it is helpful to have some understanding of the principles and concepts held by many self-actualising leaders, scientists, explorers, writers, and philosophers which have been shared since the beginning of time.

These principles have nothing to do as such with religion, but everything to do with the reality of our world and our individual potential. Such understanding builds our confidence, generates persistence, and guides our behaviour. It gives us access to the higher, unseen, and creational properties of this universe we inhabit.

Our attitudinal address is a key to our success in developing our sensitivity to higher things. Essentially, we can take one of two paths:

- We can, as adults, have a child-like attitude that wants this, or that but is not willing to do much more than shout about it. It is as though we are shouting, 'I want chocolate, I want chocolate' and hope that somehow the universe we inhabit will produce the goods like an indulgent parent.
- The second approach requires you to be a willing participant in the journey. This is holding a more mature, more active, a more participatory approach that says 'I am willing to do whatever it takes. I will release whatever is not supporting me, whether habits, friendships or unhealthy patterns of behaviour and so work to change who I am, to fulfil my potential.'

'For as a man thinks so he is.'[72]

Take a moment to:

Identify one limiting belief or thought pattern that might be holding you back.

- What evidence do you have that this belief is not entirely true?
- What would be a more empowering or realistic way of looking at the situation?

---

[72] The book of Proverbs Chapter 23 verse 7

CHAPTER 6

Quantum Physics - Mysticism or Science or ...?

Every great advance in science has issued from a new audacity of imagination.[73]

IN THE LAST CHAPTERS WE raised the seemingly mystical - that is the possibility of changing our inner world and so changing our external reality.

This is a bit like a caterpillar being released from the pupa of its past, to become free to be the butterfly that God intended it to be. I recognise such thoughts may sound a bit airy fairy; however, underlying this supposition and comprising the focal point of this chapter is Quantum Theory.

Quantum Theory shows through its many applications that our world exists in a probabilistic, and not a deterministic, dimension. What

---

[73] John Dewey, 'The Quest for Certainty', 1929

happens to us is not inevitable. The rules we rely on in our everyday lives break down.

Quantum Theory (Quantum Physics) highlights that all matter is essentially composed of energy. It ties our inner world to the outer world in ways that had not been imagined or understood by previous generations.

This, and the ensuing chapters, reflect on the science of Quantum Physics, neuroplasticity, human design, and the nature of the creation, to demonstrate the way the unseen world impacts us and how we can take advantage of the unseen world.

In truth, some of the world's recent mathematical and scientific revelations expressed through Quantum Physics and Chaos Theory can sound mystical - revelations that go far beyond common sense.

In C.S. Lewis's book, *That Hideous Strength*, the magician Merlin, advisor in King Arthur's court, was described as '*the last vestige of an old order in which matter and spirit were, from our modern point of view, confused*'. For after him came our scientific rationalist world that depended on the five senses (sight, taste, hearing, touch, smell) to determine what is possible. '*After him came the modern man to whom Nature is something dead – a machine to be worked, and to be taken to bits if it won't work the way he pleases.*'[74]

Merlin should have stuck around for a few more centuries. In the closing decades of the 20th century there arose a new mysticism, a mysticism of quarks, of neutrons, of different futures - in fact, a future defined by our growing understanding of Quantum Physics.

---

[74] Sacred Tribes retrieved 17 July 2007 from http://www.sacredtribes.com/issue2/STJ-finals/lewis-grahame-paganism.pdf

What is unusual is that while inventions such as MRI machines, computer chips, atomic clocks and lasers all depend on an understanding of quantum concepts, and physicists know how to use the equations of quantum mechanics to predict all kinds of things, it remains little understood. Caltech physicist Sean Carrol, says: *'quantum physicists are like people with iPhones; they know how to use them and can do some great things with them; but if you ask what's going on inside their iPhone, they have no idea.'*

This hasn't stopped speculation as to what mechanisms are at play – these mechanisms are known as 'interpretations'. Two of the most accepted are the Copenhagen Interpretation and the Many-Worlds Interpretation (MWI) which I will address towards the end of this chapter.

A key issue scientists face lies in the fact that the position, spin and momentum of any quantum particle is unknown until it's measured. The particle is in many states at once – it's not here or there; instead, it's here AND there, at the same time. This sounds crazy and does not fit with our world view – so how do we explain it?

In a sense, Merlin represents what we've got to get back to, albeit differently.

Quantum Physics tells us we live in a participatory universe; a universe where we now know that we are not passive beings but change makers. This is because Quantum Physics tells us that the very act of observation changes the observed. It suggests that what we do with our consciousness impacts our surroundings.

> **"No phenomenon is a real phenomenon until it is an observed phenomenon."**
> J. Wheeler

So, as the physicist John Wheeler said, 'the old word 'observer' simply must be crossed off the books, and we must put in the new word 'participator'. In this way we've come to realise that the universe is a participatory universe'.[75]

Nothing is fixed or stable and all things are in constant transition from one state to another, so we need to abandon our preconceived notions of reality and recognise that we are both the observer of our own reality and the participant in it. We both impact and create our own reality.

The strange world of Quantum Physics

'You can "dance" with the illusions of time and space, choosing your "steps" based upon things and events as they now are, or you can dance with your dreams, choosing your "steps" based upon things and events as they will be.' (Unknown).

In looking at the strange world of Quantum Physics, this chapter also backgrounds a universe of possibilities as opposed to certainties. Some of the conundrums of these possibilities are well illustrated in the following menu of Quantum Theory 'dishes':

---

[75] 'Physics, Buddhism and postmodern interpretation' *Journal of Religion and Science* Vol. 21 Issue 3 pp 287-296

> MENU[76]
>
> Our consciousness affects the behaviour of subatomic particles
>
> ....
>
> Particles move backwards as well as forwards in time and appear in all possible places at once; they are not here OR there, they are here AND there
>
> ....
>
> The universe is splitting, into billions of parallel universes[77]
>
> ....
>
> The universe is interconnected with faster-than-light transfers of information
>
> ....
>
> Coffee or Tea

These are but some of the 'dishes' on our quantum plate. Others include:

- The many parallel worlds that we can exist in, with their many different possible futures.
- At one level of existence, we, and everything around us are made up of interacting energy-fields.
- The fact that 'time' is not all it seems to be.
- Quantum entanglement shows that two particles can be separated by vast distances and somehow are connected; that

---

[76] Higgo, J, 1999 A lazy layman's guide to quantum physics retrieved 7 April 2010 from http://www.higgo.com/quantum/laymans.htm

[77] every Planck-time (10 E-43 seconds)

manipulation of one particle causes a reaction in the other, instantaneously.

- 'Empty spaces' within and between atoms are so full of energy that an area the size of a marble contains more energy than all the solid matter in the known universe.[78]

A universe for every possibility?

There is no reality in the absence of observation.[79]

Our life sits in a pathway of many possibilities. How do we best achieve what we want out of those possibilities? Can we change and attract what we want into our lives? Quantum science is increasingly affirming that we can, and we do.

Firstly, we give form to what we focus on. As noted earlier and outlined below, Quantum Theory and the double-slit experiment[80] demonstrates that an observer impacts the observed. The particle of light bubbles into our sensory world once observed. This suggests that particles have multiple possibilities. This implies that our consciousness is as important as both mass and energy.

Quantum entanglement – spooky action at a distance (Einstein)

[78] *The Clemmer Group,* 'Quantum Mechanics: Now what's the Real World? Retrieved 7 April 2010 from http://www.jimclemmer.com/blog/?p=933

[79] The Copenhagen Interpretation of Quantum Mechanics

[80] An interesting paper on this experiment and the implications for what is real can be found athttp://www4.ncsu.edu/unity/lockers/users/f/felder/public/kenny/papers/quantum.html

The paper is too long to discuss here, but seeks to explore this experiment against prevailing scientific theories culminating in the Copenhagen Interpretation of quantum mechanics.

Secondly, there is amazingly, under some circumstances, a quantum state that can be created which gives particles strange telepathic links and allows them to influence each other's properties[81]. This aspect of Quantum Physics is one that was first noted by a number of eminent scientists, including Schrodinger, Einstein, Podolsky and Rosen, and is known as 'quantum entanglement'[82]. Einstein labelled it 'spooky action at a distance'. A pair of entangled particles have an unbreakable link. When separated by vast distances, the particles will remain in the same state as each other. If you manipulate one particle, the same thing happens to the other.

It's as if the same particle exists in two different locations at once.

This concept has played a very important role in Quantum Information Theory and the foundations of Quantum Mechanics. It has clear implications for all of our lives. It's considered to be one of the deepest aspects of Quantum Mechanics. The concept of quantum entanglement is central in the development of quantum teleportation[83], quantum cryptography[84] and the quantum computer.

---

[81] The Science Show Retrieved 1 October 2008 from http://www.abc.net.au/rn/scienceshow/stories/2008/2190074.htm

[82] Even Einstein had difficulties in coming to grips with what Quantum Entanglement is about. As Duncan McKimm put it: *Quantum entanglement is an area of science that will one day dominate the way we look at information, the way we communicate secretly and the way our computers do their thing. Problem is, it's really bloody confusing.* I recommend you Google it.

[83] Quantum teleportation provides a mechanism of moving a quantum bit or qubit from one location to another, without having to physically transport the underlying particle that a qubit is normally attached to. Much like the invention of the telegraph allowed classical bits to be transported at high speed across continents, quantum teleportation holds the promise that one day, qubits could be moved likewise.

[84] Quantum cryptography uses our current knowledge of physics to develop a cryptosystem that is not able to be defeated - that is, one that is completely secure against being compromised without knowledge of the sender or the receiver of the messages

Although quantum entanglement is very fundamental and useful, it is also mysterious. In one quantum entanglement experiment with light, which has the overtones of a Star Trek '*beam me up Scotty*' transporter, a phenomenon was uncovered in an intriguing demonstration that was carried out in 1998 at the California Institute of Technology and at Aarhus University in Denmark.[85]

> **Everything in our universe is interconnected. The universe is "a sea of energy" and we all are part of this sea.**

The researchers there investigated the phenomena of the entanglement of light particles at a subatomic level. Entanglement of light occurs when two photons of light have related properties even when they are far apart. In fact, their properties are so entwined that information in one is correlated in the other.

> **The day science begins to study non-physical phenomena it will make more progress than in all the previous centuries of existence.**
> (N.Tesla 1856 -1943 inventor of alternating current, violet ray, neon light, and holder of 275 other patents)

If you do something to one photon, then *instantaneously* the other will change. This seemingly breaks the law which says nothing can happen faster than the speed of light. The scientists in this experiment then used two entangled beams to carry information about the state of a third beam. '*In a sense they have created a replica of the original light beam. What has been transmitted from one light beam to another is information that was used to recreate the original beam.*'[86]

---

[85] BBC news Retrieved 2 February 2008 from http://news.bbc.co.uk/2/hi/science/nature/201815.stm

[86] Ibid

This is your Star Trek transporter.

This experiment suggests that below the surface of our conscious reality there is a deeply interlinked web of interaction that permeates our universe whose parameters are still largely unknown. It also suggests to us that the universe that we inhabit is an integrated whole and is one that cannot be understood simply by analysis – the whole is greater than the sum of its parts. Systems theory seen on a quantum scale.

I mention these things to highlight that Quantum Physics raises many scientific and philosophical issues that are unresolved. The experiments in these and other areas ask many questions that demand a. framework of understanding – an explanatory interpretation of the theory, if you like.

Recognising the implications of these facets of quantum science will help us understand the rationale behind The IDEA.

Few of us, however, are going to be excited by the mathematical modelling of Quantum Physics. What we do want to know is how the concepts might have an impact on us. What are the implications for our lives and our journey? It is in that spirit that this section is written.

What was originally called Quantum Mechanics is now also known as Quantum Physics, and Quantum Theory. Quantum Mechanics was so called as it superseded the theory of Newtonian mechanics. *'In the Newtonian world view, everything is one vast machine or mechanism made up of matter and energy. This machine is entirely deterministic which means that if you knew the speed and position of every piece of matter in the universe you would know its entire future — just as if you knew the speed and position of the balls on a billiard table, you could calculate where they will all end up. Everything happens (time moves forward) in a three-dimensional space. Consciousness and mind have absolutely no place in this model; they are not on the map'.* [87]

> **In Quantum Physics the very act of watching affects the observed reality**

Our civilisation's thinking on the nature of reality has been largely formed by the science and philosophy of Newtonian mechanics. This is because the principles seem to work well enough; after all the planets are still orbiting as predicted by Newtonian physics. Newtonian physics does, however, imply a certain lack of personal control over our lives and our destiny as cause and effect follow a linear pathway.

By contrast, Quantum Theory presents a staggeringly different picture of our world. In Quantum Theory, the world exists in a sea of possibility and probability. Recognising this, the scientific world has acknowledged that the result of a process or measurement can only be predicted with a level of probability, even if it is a very high probability. This means that scientific laws are probabilistic, not as once thought deterministic. Nothing is certain. As mentioned previously, Newtonian mechanics says that if you throw a rubber ball at a wall it will bounce back. Quantum Theory says that there is a possibility, however remote, that it will go through the wall in an effect known as tunneling. This principle has been used by Samsung in a mobile phone component which it sells to several handset manufacturers and now has licensed as the Quantum Tunneling Composite (QTC). Once again, reality can prove stranger than fiction and the resulting technology will become integrated in a raft of new devices.

---

[87] EnergyGrid Retrieved 1 February 2008 from http://www.energygrid.com/science/2004/12ap-quantummap.html

In Quantum Physics everything is moving in multiple dimensions, including parallel universes. Time is simply another dimension and time becomes relative, as Einstein[88] pointed out, and it only appears to be moving forward. Philosophically, space and time cannot be separated. Nothing is certain – even looking at something is significant. In fact, one of the most well-known Quantum Physics statements, *'Observation changes the observed'*, is grounded in a repeatable scientific experiment. This is sometimes known as the 'observer effect'. Taking it one step further, if something is going to be measured, then 'the measurement process can fundamentally alter what is being measured'.[89] This is extraordinary and is hard to understand but forces us to change our view of reality.

The philosophical understandings about the nature of *reality* and *being* remain largely embedded in the old physics of the nineteenth and early twentieth century. The different assumptions that flow out from quantum science have yet to pervade our twenty-first century culture and thinking. Perhaps this is because the paradigm shift required is so profound that developing a philosophical framework around it is too radical to gain acceptance. It requires a shift in consciousness.

In the meantime, Quantum Theory certainly works[90] in the real world. For example, we have such applications of Quantum Theory as lasers, magnetic memories, transistors, superconductors, nuclear

---

[88] Albert Einstein (14 March 1879 – 18 April 1955) was a German born theoretical physicist best known for his theory of relativity, and specifically his great insight that matter and energy are really different forms of the same thing. Matter can be turned into energy, and energy into matter, as explained in the famous equation $E = mc^2$, for which he received a Nobel Prize.

[89] Nature: International weekly journal of science, 'quantum physics: observing and the observed', 443, 154-155 (14 September 2006) | doi:10.1038/443154a; Published online 13 September 2006

[90] EnergyGrid Retrieved 1 February 2008 from http://www.energygrid.com/science/2004/12ap-quantummap.html

magnetic resonance technology (NMR) and superconducting quantum interference device (SQUID) measuring devices,[91] quantum computers, and so on. Therefore, however weird or counterintuitive quantum science may seem, it affects our daily life. Explaining it is another matter. It is useful for us to learn that this branch of science can inform us of what lies behind the reality of our possibility thinking.

Observation, the key to active participation

Observation changes our thinking and practices in life and so it is also true to say that observation changes our world. That Quantum Physics demonstrates that an observer impacts the observed is amazing to most of us. As the eminent theoretical and mathematical physicist, Pascual Jordan, said: 'Observations not only disturb what is to be measured, they produce it'.[92]

> **Observations not only disturb what is to be measured, they produce it.**

Improving our observation and our attention span are, therefore, valuable disciplines to develop.

The double-slit experiment[93] with light implies there are realms of existences that bubble into our world when observed. Light travels as both a wave and a particle. A particle of light in this experiment sits in a wave of positions. When you

[91] Measuring device having a squid magnetometer with a modulator for measuring magnetic fields of extremely low frequency

[92] https://quantumenigma.com/nutshell/notable-quotes-on-quantum-physics/

[93] An interesting paper on this experiment and the implications for what is real can be found at http://www4.ncsu.edu/unity/lockers/users/f/felder/public/kenny/papers/quantum.html

The paper is too long to discuss here but seeks to explore this experiment against prevailing scientific theories culminating in the Copenhagen Interpretation of quantum mechanics.

observe it, you effectively pull it out of a quantum soup and give it a reality and it becomes a particle. The act of observation is the act of simplifying the observed because we see the object from one angle only – a single state, for example up or down, but not up AND down simultaneously.

Related to this, many scientists now acknowledge that in a similar manner, 'the act of measurement causes the collapse of either the wave or the particle function, depending upon the system of measurement used in the experiment; only upon measurement does the potential become actual.'[94]

Unsurprisingly, the effect of observation on the observed is a problem when it comes to some real-life applications of Quantum Physics. One such application is in the realm of countering the significant trade in counterfeit currency. Counterfeit currency has been a major headache for sovereign states for as long as they have existed.

You may be familiar with the concepts of Bitcoin and cryptocurrency. Research has looked at developing a hard copy currency with some of the same features seen in Bitcoin; the currency would be called quantum money. This initiative was developed with a strong focus on defeating would-be counterfeiters of currency. It would encode the digital currency with a random binary string in a fixed secret set of bases.

This concept of quantum money has long been explored as the solution to the international trade in counterfeit notes. It overcomes counterfeiting by storing sequences of photons within banknotes, along with a serial number. The photons would be randomly polarised

---

[94] The Bridge Retrieved 16 April 2010 from http://science-spirituality.blogspot.com/2009/05/his-holiness-dalai-lama-provides.html

during printing and the bank would keep a secret record of photon polarisations for each banknote.[95] It was thought to be an answer because the moment you try to copy it the very act of observing/ measuring the photon polarisations will destroy their ability to reflect their quantum states irreversibly. They can no longer be 0 and 1 at the same time; rather they have to become one or the other.[96] The problem is that because of such peculiar qualities, only the issuing bank could verify the note and that is certainly not practical.

What this demonstrates is that because observation changes reality, reality is both external to you and internal to you. What the double-slit experiment and other applications show is that we shape and affect our experience of reality through the way the internal workings of our mind impact on our external world, by way of the simple medium of observation.

The ability to focus and maintain our attention varies from one person to another depending on a range of emotional, physical, and nutritional factors; but how well we pay attention, or observe, is important - more on this later. Unfortunately, intruding on our ability to truly observe is a gremlin. This gremlin is our increasing addiction to the external sensory world around us.

We drown ourselves in electronic sounds; immerse ourselves in electronic and print media, including television soapies, and the electronic media, such as online games, and streaming television (which has been called 'the chewing gum of the mind'); then there is all the Hollywood gossip we must catch up on, and we go on to hook ourselves up to 24/7 communication channels (mobiles, emails, social

---

[95] James Morris, 'Quantum Money', Available at: http://kerneltrap.org/node/4241. Accessed on 30 April 2010

[96] Mullins, J. 'Note Perfect', *New Scientist* 17 April 2010 p41

media, notepads, news channels, etcetera.). We then wonder why our lives are lived at an increasingly reactive, rather than a responsive, level, let alone at a creative and reflective level.

The difference between reactive and responsive levels is huge in the impact it has on our wellbeing, awareness, and ability to achieve our potential.

Reaction comes out of an emotion such as fear, anxiety, anger, and so on. Imagine your reaction to a large spider falling into your lap, or a wasp in the car that you are driving. It is the unthinking response which in some circumstances might see you unthinkingly reaching for the potato chips when hungry or the cool drink when thirsty or the television control when bored.

Responsiveness comes out of a mental assessment, a genuine awareness, that engages our pre-frontal cortex which is that part of our brain where our free will is located.

But, for evolutionary and cultural reasons, we tend to be reactive.

Our reactivity is further elevated in today's world where we input such a constant overload of information; a world where we choose to be accessible at any time to almost anyone. This creates stresses unknown in the past. This is a world where such stresses quickly make us reactive. You only have to think about the rapidly increasing phenomenon of road rage, a phenomenon that affects both genders and has seen insurance premiums rise for women in recent times as they too in the past several decades have become full participants in the connected world. [97]

---

[97] Mr Traffic Retrieved 1 December 2007 from http://www.mrtraffic.com/rage.htm

If we are, however, to impact and create our own reality, we need to be responsive and feed our creative reflective level, as will be outlined later. Locating ourselves in a constant reactive mode denies our Inner Consciousness the opportunity it needs to create pathways to a better life. By contrast, our outer consciousness responds powerfully to the sensory 24/7 world around us. Therefore, we need to control our sensory input if our lives are not going to be built on reactions.

Throughout this book the imperative, demonstrated by scientific research, is biased towards learning to respond, and not react, to the challenges that life puts in our path.

It is normal for our attention to be focussed on the world around us; however, we need also to turn inwards. We need to be aware of what is sometimes called our Inner Consciousness. Inner Consciousness is not simply the awareness of thoughts, emotions or even our physical body, but it is deeper than that. It is a higher state of mind. It is being fully aware and conscious of the sensation of being alive and all that entails.

Have you ever watched a beautiful sunset, listened to a magical piece of music, been a part of something extraordinary that has touched you so deeply that you became lost in the experience? In these moments, we can set aside our closely held beliefs and paradigms and extend the boundaries of our existence as we touch the skirts of the Universe's energy fields with awareness. We are no longer reactive; rather, we become open.

One of the values of art (painting, music, literature, etcetera) in our culture is that it is a medium that, at its best, interprets life in all its forms for us in a manner that can challenge our perspective. It can act as a prism on the light of our sensory world. It is the ultimate mirror of our existence and can enable us to become open and to respond differently to the world we find ourselves in. It is a mechanism for reaching our inner world, giving voice to our souls. It is a pathway to our Inner Consciousness.

Our Inner Consciousness is our spirit life entering our material existence. It allows the mind to transcend the boundaries of our senses, of time and space.

This leads me to the Quantum Physics world of an inter-relational unity. This is the place where beliefs shape reality. This is where our being interfaces with the unseen forces of the universe and can shatter the self-limiting paradigms we hold.

We can block our Inner Consciousness from working in our lives by creating a sensory overload of electronic media. This is not what our design features are about. While the Creator has given us the free will to make the most of love and life, we can create meaninglessness, despair, and sadness by saturating ourselves in the cotton wool of sensory input and choosing not to be aware of life beyond our physical senses, in our daily living.

> **Quantum Physics is a world of an inter-relational unity. This is the place where beliefs shape reality. This is where our being interfaces with the unseen forces of the universe and can shatter the self-limiting paradigms we hold.**

We have a choice, a decision. The choice is ours, is yours, it is mine! We need to consciously undertake daily practices that create the outcomes we seek.

So, let us free ourselves to some degree from being engaged 24/7 with the material world around us. Switch off for at least twelve hours a day our smart phones with all their applications, our televisions, computers, mobiles and notepads. Let's limit our time on Facebook, Twitter, Tik Tok, or other networking sites, and choose love and life. In this way, we provide space to creatively shatter those paradigms of false limits created by the electronic media we daily bathe in.

Let us give our being creative space. We must take responsibility for what happens in our lives.

The two leading interpretations to explain Quantum Physics:

Such explanations of Quantum Theory, as outlined below, help us understand our world better. These explanations, known as 'interpretations', also help explain why our beliefs begin to define our individual reality. The two most accepted interpretations are:

- the Copenhagen Interpretation; and
- the Many-Worlds Interpretation (MWI).

The Copenhagen Interpretation

The first major attempt at an explanation acceptable to most scientists was known as The Copenhagen Interpretation. The Copenhagen Interpretation is a collection of views principally attributed to Niels Bohr and Werner Heisenberg. It is one of the oldest of numerous proposed interpretations of Quantum Theory, as features of it date to the development of Quantum Mechanics during 1925–1927.

In summary, The Copenhagen Interpretation makes a distinction between the observer and the observed; when no one is watching, a system evolves deterministically according to a wave equation, but when someone is watching, the wave function of the system collapses to the observed state, which is why the act of observing changes the system.[98]

The Copenhagen Interpretation remains a popular basis of understanding Quantum Physics, perhaps because of its simplicity.

While answering some questions raised by Quantum Theory, the perceived problem with the Copenhagen Interpretation lies in the unique status accorded to the observer which is not given to any other aspect of the theory, nor does it explain the observer. However, in 1957 an American physicist, Dr Hugh Everett III proposed a different theory that overcame this and other puzzles that Quantum Mechanics posed. This approach is known as the Many-Worlds Interpretation.

Many-Worlds Interpretation
This is a 'mind-blowing' interpretation, but one which enjoys strong support.

The Many-Worlds Interpretation sought to address the anomalies thrown up by other interpretations, not least the Copenhagen Interpretation, but in doing so it poses some real challenges to the way we see and understand our world.

According to this interpretation, our future being exists in different worlds of different possibilities.

Whenever numerous viable possibilities exist, the world splits into many worlds, one world for each different possibility (in this context, the term 'worlds' refers to what most people call 'universes'). In each of these worlds, everything is identical, except for that one different choice; [once the choice

---

[98] The Many-Worlds Interpretation of Quantum Mechanics Retrieved 27 May 207 from http://www.station1.net/DouglasJones/many.htm

is made] from that point on, the 'worlds' develop independently, and no communication is possible between them, so the people living in those worlds (and splitting along with them) may have no idea that this is going on. In this way, the world branches endlessly. What is 'the present' to us lies in the pasts of an unaccountably huge number of different futures. Everything that can *happen, does, somewhere.*[99]

The Many-Worlds Interpretation does seem a little crazy, but Quantum Physics already seems a bit bizarre and, interestingly, while there is no consensus the Many-Worlds approach is one of the top three most popular ways to make sense of what's going on, according to surveys of relevant experts.

Where the Copenhagen Interpretation attempts to explain what appears to be a 'wave function' collapse when a particle is observed, the Many-Worlds Interpretation says that there is no collapse; rather, it's a splitting of world. This, in quantum speak, is known as 'decoherence'.

Many people will find the Many-Worlds Interpretation, and the consequences that flow from it, deeply disturbing because it is counter-intuitive and radically alters our sense of place in the physical world. Such discomfort exists amongst a great many physicists as noted below. It is also apparent that a large number of physicists, including many who *teach* physics, do not have a good understanding of the Many-Worlds Interpretation.[100]

Polls taken among quantum theorists have, however, revealed that most of them nonetheless believe that the Many-Worlds Interpretation

[99] Jones, D.S. Retrieved 10 January 2008 from http://www.station1.net/DouglasJones/many.htm

[100] The Many-Worlds Interpretation of Quantum Mechanics Retrieved 2 February 2008 from http://www.station1.net/DouglasJones/many.htm

represents, in some sense, an accurate description of the way the world really is.

One such poll was conducted in the 1980s by the political scientist David Raub. Amongst the many supporters of the Many-Worlds Interpretation were such notables as Stephen Hawking and Nobel Laureates Murray Gell-Mann and Richard Feynman. Gell-Mann and Hawking recorded reservations with the name *many-worlds*, but not with the theory's content. Nobel Laureate Steven Weinberg is also mentioned as a 'many-worlder'.[101]

Unsurprisingly, the polls also show that many of these scientists would rather not discuss the subject.[102] Doubtless this is because, as mentioned above, the implications are broader than our current understanding of reality permits.

Scientific theory has advanced to the point where, like it or hate it, the concept of parallel universes is accepted – and many scientists, whilst acknowledging the reality of the science, hate the idea as it is such an uncomfortable concept. This is because the idea of parallel universes, as outlined, suggests that there is one universe for every possibility.

But the days when scientists could ignore the idea of parallel universes are gone forever. In fact, 'David Deutsch at the University of Oxford has shown that the key equations of quantum mechanics arise from the mathematics of parallel universes. 'This work will go down as one of the most important developments in the history of science' says Andy Albrecht, a physicist at the University of California.'[103]

----

[101] The Everett FAQ Retrieved 2 February 2008 from http://www.hedweb.com/manworld.htm#believes

[102] Jones, D.S. Retrieved 10 January 2008 from http://www.station1.net/DouglasJones/many.htm

[103] Merali, Z. 2007 'Parallel Universes are born again' *New Scientist Vol. 195* No 2622 22 September 2007 pp6-7

The idea of Parallel Universes has been around for over 50 years, when it was first proposed by Hugh Everett at Princeton, and now leads to a Many Worlds scenario known as the multiverse[104] in the broader scientific community.

This brief description of the Many-Worlds Interpretation is clearly not rigorous but is a taster to encourage you to explore the concept further at your own leisure.

Finally, even though we have only lightly reviewed some applications of Quantum Physics in this chapter, it will be evident that quantum superpositions,[105] and the resulting quantum technologies, are only just beginning to make an impact, but the impact is such that that with new advances in silicon it is only a matter of time before it becomes more part of our everyday lives.

---

[104] The Many-Worlds Interpretation of Quantum Mechanics Retrieved 27 May 207 from http://www.station1.net/DouglasJones/many.htm

[105] Superposition is a principle of Quantum Theory that describes a challenging concept about the nature and behavior of matter and forces at the sub-atomic level. The principle of superposition claims that while we do not know what the state of any object is, it is actually in all possible states simultaneously, as long as we don't look to check. It is the measurement itself that causes the object to be limited to a single possibility.

CHAPTER 7

Synchronicity and the Law of Attraction

'The great Swiss psychologist, CG Jung, defines 'synchronicity' as a meaningful coincidence.'[106]

Synchronicity and 'clairknowing'[107]

LIKE QUANTUM PHYSICS, SYNCHRONICITY CHALLENGES the idea of a separation between space, time, and the different material objects in this universe. Synchronicity is an affront to the Newtonian rationalist scientific paradigm of our world, with the Newtonian marginalisation of the unseen in a dualistic interpretation of life that alienates us from the natural world around us.

---

[106] Google definitions Retrieved 19 April 2008 from http://www.google.com.au/search?num=100&hl=en&lr=lang_en&safe=active&defl=en&q=define:Synchronicity&sa=X&oi=glossary_definition&ct=title

[107] Clairknowing is a term that I think embraces the times where you just 'know' something in the future in a way that is not quite clairvoyance but is more than intuition.

In a Jungian sense, synchronous events are those things, people, or events that you attract into your life in an inexplicable manner. Such a coincidence of events, however 'seems to be meaningfully related and is conceived in Jungian theory as an explanatory principle on the same order as causality.'[108] Causality being the relationship between cause and effect.

Synchronicity carries many of the undertones of the Law of Attraction which says that you create your reality whether you are aware of it or not. The Law of Attraction is discussed later in this chapter.

Probably one of the most common examples of synchronicity is finding a parking space just when we need one. How many of us end up some place where parking is an issue? Despite knowing in our conscious mind that we are unlikely to find a parking space, we still drive down the street and suddenly a car pulls out, or miraculously there is a space. That is a small example of synchronicity. Or perhaps, we are thinking of someone and the phone rings and there they are on the end of the phone, or, thinking about a particular problem, and then randomly encountering information or a person who provides a solution.

Now try doing it with your conscious mind (visualise it) and watch how your hit rate increases – that is the Law of Attraction at work.

Synchronicity is premised on the fact that matter and the unconscious mind interpenetrate.

Personally, one of the most awful examples of synchronicity that occurred to me took place some years ago. I was running a charity, and times were tough. I had to let go a senior manager who I

---

[108] The Free Dictionary Retrieved 20 April 2008 from http://www.thefreediction-ary.com/synchronicity

personally held dear and who was a major asset to the charity. As I was breaking the news to her, a wren flew into the window and, to the horror of us both, broke its neck. It was a visual illustration of the small death that was about to occur in that room that morning.

Synchronicity is premised on the fact that matter and the unconscious mind interpenetrate. This is an underpinning premise in The IDEA, one that defines this book and one that finds an echo in Quantum Physics. Synchronicity is conceptually older than Jung's description of causality and finds its roots in the philosophers of the sixteenth and seventeenth centuries. It is experienced at many levels of our being far more frequently than you could or would ever know if you are living an unconscious (unaware) life.

In a remarkable example of so-called coincidence or synchronicity, mathematician Warren Weaver in his book, *Lady Luck: the Theory of Probability*, recounts the fascinating tale of coincidence that stretches our traditional notions of chance to their breaking point. The story originally appeared in *Life* Magazine.

Weaver writes:

> *'All fifteen members of a church choir in Beatrice, Nebraska, due at practice at 7:20 were late on the evening of March 1 1950. The minister, his wife and daughter had one reason (the wife delayed to iron the daughters dress); one girl waited until she had finished a geometry problem; one could not start her car; two lingered to hear the end of an especially exciting radio program; one mother and daughter were late because the mother had to call the daughter twice to wake her from a nap, and so on. The reasons seemed rather ordinary. But there were ten separate and unconnected reasons for the lateness of fifteen persons. It was rather fortunate that none of the fifteen arrived on time at 7:20 for at 7:25 the*

building was destroyed in an explosion. The members of the choir,
Life reported, wondered if their delay was 'an act of God.' [109]

When we become aware of them, such synchronous events encourage us on life's road as they suggest a life hidden from our realm and operating in the unseen, giving us hope. Indeed, synchronicity is significant as it appears to demonstrate a collective unconscious or what Hungarian-born writer, Arthur Koestler, states as the *'fundamental unity of all things, which transcends mechanical causality, and which relates coincidence to the universal scheme of things.'* [110]

The universal mind is a concept with many shades of meaning, from that of Jung's conception of the Collective Unconscious, to a broader meaning of the interpenetrating sum total of the minds of all sentient beings in all time-spaces. [111] Its nature is experienced at the rim of our reality and, if we are open, then our lives are affected accordingly. Let me give you another example, this time of an incident that occurred recently in a good friend's life.

Sarah (not her real name) had gone to the public swimming pool complex with her two children and her partner. Whilst the children had their swimming classes, she swam her laps. The children's classes finished and their father took the two girls to the water play area whilst Sarah continued her laps. Coming to her last lap, she felt the strongest impulse to swim across two lanes and do her last lap in a totally different lane. Being open to what her intuition told her, she

---

[109] The Mystery of Chance, Retrieved 20 April 2008 from http://www.strangemag.com/mysteryofchance.html

[110] Communiversity Magazine Retrieved 20 April 2008 from http://www.communiversitymagazine.org/web%20pages/Our%20Place%20in%20the%20Universe.htm

[111] Library of the hidden estate, Retrieved 24 March 2008 from http://www.sakara.net/Mind.html

swam across the two lanes to get to where she felt she had to go. As she swam across these lanes, she saw what she thought was her daughter's earring at the bottom of the pool. Recovering it, she went to her daughter and sure enough, she had lost it whilst completing her classes.

How did that happen? I am sure that you know of, or have perhaps experienced, situations like this which can only be explained in terms of the greater consciousness of the universe around us; a consciousness with which our own minds are intertwined; however, we tend to live our lives unconscious of that greater consciousness. When we are open, conscious, and aware of this, then we are drawn into action, circumstances and coincidences that allow thoughts to materialise and shape a reality.

This isn't wishful thinking; it's the way things have always been in time and space. Synchronicity is seemingly the crystallisation, in the physical realm, of processes that find their origin in the unseen. As such it is another dimension, if not an overlapping one of the Law of Attraction.

This interpenetration of all things, both seen and unseen, is also reflective of Quantum Physics and Chaos Theory. Both theories highlight the lattices of connection which result in the isolation and separation experienced in the material world being more apparent than real.

As Alexander Pope [112] three hundred years ago put it:

---

[112] Alexander Pope (1688 –1744) is generally regarded as the greatest English poet of the eighteenth century.

'Nothing is foreign; parts relate to whole;
One all-extending, all-preserving soul
Connects each being,
Greatest with the least.' [113]

We have previously discussed the paradigms of existence that we hold to be true. Such paradigms are based on our experience of life as discovered through our five physical senses - touch, taste, smell, hearing and sight. Such paradigms give us a bounded sense of who we are in the physical world we inhabit and lead us to make assumptions on causality. These assumptions relate to the nature of time, of past, present and future, and of the nature of matter and energy. What synchronicity tells us is that many of the distinctions arising out of these and other assumptions are not found in absolute truths but are matters of our own perception.

The Jung scholar Dr. Roderick Main writes extensively on synchronicity and its wider implications in his book *The Rupture of Time*. He writes:

'Synchronicity suggests that there are uncaused events, that matter has a psychic aspect, that the psyche can relativise time and space, and that there may be a dimension of objective meaning accessible to but not created by humans. If the psyche can relativise time and space, then it becomes possible for temporally and spatially distant events somehow to involve themselves in the here and now without any normal channel of causal transmission. If there is a dimension of objective meaning, this implies that the meaning we experience is not always or entirely our subjective creation, individually or as a species, but that we may be woven into an order of meaning that transcends our human perspective.' [114]

---

[113] About.com Classic literature, Retrieved 20 April from http://classiclit.about.com/library/bl-etexts/apope/bl-apope-essay-3.htm
[114] Main, R. 2004 The rupture of time: synchronicity and Jung's critique of modern Western culture Published by Brunner-Routledge UK

In an example of how the psyche can relativise time and space, my wife had a 'clairknowing'[115] event some years ago when standing on the platform at Gravesend station in England waiting to catch the 7:29 morning train to Charing Cross Station. She waited in her usual spot to get into the front carriage; however, as she heard the train approaching, she experienced a deep sense of unease that grew into such a fear that by the time the train pulled to a stop she could not get onto it. Having missed that train, she subsequently heard that three stations later the train's front carriage derailed, with many passengers suffering injury. Space and time were relativised and what was a future event was sensed in the present.

In another example, a friend of mine's grand-mum had a similar experience as she waited to board a ship in Estonia ahead of the Russian advance during the Second World War. You could only imagine her anxiety to take herself and her children away from the frontline of a war and a vengeful army. She had waited for hours and hours on the quayside and then, just as she approached the gangplank, she changed her mind due to a strong inner urging. The ship sailed without her and was bombed a short time later. All on board perished. Fortunately, she was able to later leave Estonia by another vessel.

Again, there was a relativisation of space/time that created a synchronous event in which the individual was perceptive enough to discern or intuit a reality that is continuous and united, in ways that are both visible and invisible, both seen and unseen.

---

[115] Clairknowing is a term that I think embraces the times where you just 'know' something in the future in a way that is not quite clairvoyance.

Chaos Theory

'Just as quantum physics demonstrates a participatory universe, chaos theory demonstrates the power of that participation.

This realisation of interconnectivity has generated a broadening of scientific paradigms and the development of new theories, such as those of Quantum Physics, Systems Theory, the Theory of Relativity and Chaos Theory.

Chaos Theory recognises the interconnectivity of all things. It suggests the existence of an underlying order in the midst of apparent disorder. The name of the Theory almost gives lie to its content. It holds that small changes in initial conditions can result in vast changes in the outcomes. In a popularised example it suggests that a butterfly flapping its wings in Brazil can, through the tiny change it makes in the atmosphere, subsequently contribute to the actual creation of a hurricane in Florida a year or two later. Those things we take for granted around us are, therefore, always on the edge of sudden and radical change, impacted by unknown, often seemingly insignificant, connected, events occurring in the fabric of our ecosystem.

In the same way as we work to change our thinking and actions, however incrementally, we place ourselves in the arena of possible sudden and radical change. In this way, we change our world. Authentic spirituality starts in an awareness of who we are in this creative act. Just as Quantum Physics demonstrates a participatory universe, Chaos Theory demonstrates the power of that participation.

I came across a lovely clarification of what this means on the Internet recently. I quote an excerpt here:

'The process of spirituality is the process of becoming conscious in all areas of our lives. We meditate, for example, so that we can be awake in mental states in which most are unconscious — i.e. those states with minimal and/or predictable/boring sensory input (we even eventually become conscious in our sleep); we forgive our enemies because we do not want to be unconsciously blinded by anger and resentment; we enjoy helping others because of a growing awareness of our collective nature; we do yoga so that we become more conscious of our body/mind; we analyse our dreams and fantasies, so that we may become conscious of psyche and the disowned parts of ourselves; and we become more mindful of our thinking so that we can consciously direct our mind's reality-creation and or filtering processes, and to realise how contrived most of our beliefs about reality actually are. So, spirituality can be considered the movement towards ever greater consciousness in all aspects of our lives.[116]

This awareness allows us to remain open to 'spiritual experiences' outside of the established framework of our faith system, be it Buddhism, Christianity, or any other faith system. This is possible because we become increasingly aware of the unseen aspects of creation.

Of course, to be open and aware of such things as synchronous events and all that they might imply about the nature of the universe, means our beliefs have to be open to the possibility that we are more than individuals locked in space and time walking a predetermined and solitary journey through the time allotted to our existence.

Understand that knowledge of synchronicity helps us to appreciate the interconnection of all things. We gain from it an ecological perspective

---

[116] EnergyGrid Retrieved 20 February 2008 from
http://energygrid.com/spirit/2007/05ap-beconscious.html

of our universe. From this derives Jung's notion of causality (That is to say, how one event causes another).

In parallel with synchronicity is the concept of intuition. Intuition is caught up with undertones of precognition and clairvoyance – or *words of knowledge* as the Bible puts it. It is seen by many of various beliefs to have spiritual connotations. Yet, that inner knowing is reflected in a Jungian understanding of synchronicity, as touched on earlier.

Was it intuition that saved my wife from a train wreck, or synchronicity? The lines between the two are blurred and beside the point. The point is – are we open and aware? Are we living consciously? This is important because, if you are, then research indicates a greater ability to draw on these facets of creation to our advantage. It is no different to the Law of Attraction. Creation will go on without our consciously playing a role; the Universe will still respond to us because of our interconnectedness, but if we choose to be aware and play a conscious role, then how we choose to change our world will be to our benefit.

The simple truth is that each day our lives encounter meaningful coincidences or synchronicities that we have attracted into them.

The Law of Attraction

'All the truths about life are not secrets, but they are hidden from us due to our ignorance.' (Author unknown)

We have talked about the concept of the Universal Mind when discussing synchronicity. Parallel to that concept is the notion that the universe is also composed of different energy fields, including that energy which I would call spiritual energy. Such energy fields flow throughout the universe, waiting to be aligned by external factors.

And there is more … As previously discussed, the universe is also governed by many different natural laws which shape the way that these energy fields are aligned with each other and with the material world, not least with you and me.

Some of these laws (such as gravity) are more obvious than others. Another of the laws is the so-called Law of Attraction.

At its simplest, the Law of Attraction says that *energy will attract like energy*. Another way of putting it is that everything draws to itself that which is like it. This happens through the energy fields of the universe. All living things have an energy field or an energy envelope around them that is measurable.

Your brain is comprised of a tight network of nerve cells, all interacting with one another and generating an overall electrical field. In earlier chapters we noted that consciousness is the key to making the mysteries of quantum mechanics work because the one difference between us and a photon is that we can think, we are conscious. As such, we can choose which of the possibilities before us to collapse our wave function into.

The mind affects the frequency in the energy field.

It is our beliefs that give an emotional quality to our thoughts, and that emotional quality has much more power to create a perceivable reality than our thoughts alone. Therefore, we will attract those things into our lives that our minds think most about and are the most emotive about.

Another way of putting it is that *what you focus on expands*. The concept is well known and has been known for centuries. In his best-selling book *Think and Grow Rich*, Napoleon Hill makes the statement *Truly, thoughts are things, and powerful things at that when mixed with definiteness of purpose, persistence, and burning desire for their translation into riches or other objects.*[117]

The science as to why this happens is outlined throughout this book and finds its context in the philosophical position it takes.

Like all the Laws of the universe, the Law of Attraction, which forms the premise of Napoleon Hill's statement, is undiscriminating. This is because the created universe (unlike the Creator) is essentially indifferent. Its Laws apply regardless of whether you consciously focus your thoughts or, unconsciously but emotionally, project them as you go about your daily life being happy, fearful, or anxious.

If the Law of Attraction works regardless of whether we are consciously or unconsciously shaping our world through our thinking, then being conscious about our thought processes is literally life changing. All emotionally loaded thoughts influence material outcomes. We live in a universe of energy, and as we will learn, this energy is vibrational. Consequently, *feeling-thoughts* set up a scientifically demonstrable frequency which becomes the cause of its own effect.

Whether that frequency generates good things or bad things is our responsibility. When our focus is on the things or situations that we desire, we meet the criteria for the Law. Unfortunately, this is also the case if our focus is on the things we do not want or desire. In that instance we also begin to fulfil the Law, because in both cases it is to do with where our attention (or our thoughts) is focussed. The Law is indiscriminate.

The conclusion we can draw is that if we don't want something, then 'don't give it so much of our time and emotions'.

---

[117] Hill, N., 1937 Think and grow rich, Filiquarian Publishing LLC p19

Make sense?

Therefore, living consciously and being aware becomes so important, so that we can then gate-keep our thinking. There are exercises at the end of this book which will help you along your journey, should you undertake them.

Living consciously starts with self-awareness. It is out of our inner being that our stream of consciousness arises. Meditation helps us become more self-aware; in particular, meditations that invoke insight, such as Mindfulness Meditation.

Feeling-thoughts set up a scientifically demonstrable frequency which becomes the cause of its own effect.

As discussed in earlier chapters, your inner world will, and does, create your outer world, as we will also see in the Law of Correspondence. You have it within your power to create the life that you consciously desire.

It can all seem so simple really – just think it and it appears – a bit like that program of *Bewitched* which recounts the story of Samantha who with a twitch of her nose just manifested the new reality. Fortunately, it is not so easy and working consciously with the Law of Attraction takes time and requires focus and desire.

Why fortunately? Well, because we also tend to do a lot of negative *what if* pitches to the universe (what if I lost my job, money, health, a child, etcetera) and the accumulated effect of these would rapidly turn into a negative reality were it not for the safety fuses that apply and one of those 'fuses' is the need for persistence.

The need for persistence

One of the major problems that people have in getting the most out of the Law of Attraction is a lack of persistence. As individuals many of us suffer from a real difficulty in being persistent. We can become easily distracted.

We start diets and slowly they fade away (even as we do not); we give up smoking / vaping, again and again; we commit to exercising, but our routines become fractured; we promise ourselves that we will study harder to improve ourselves, but our work days consume us; New Year's resolutions are made every year and every year they evaporate in the warmth of the summer sun; and so it goes on. We give up too easily if we don't see the outcome within days or hours or even minutes of pitching our dream. When it comes to the Law of Attraction, we need to be persistent.

The whole secret of not slipping from success to failure is to never take our eyes off the ball. Successful people will know that when they fail, it is as often as not because their focus shifted and they stopped paying attention to the game.

Our mind does not maintain an unconscious focus. We must remain aware. We must maintain conscious mental control. If we control our thoughts, we will control our circumstances.

Everything is created first in the unseen and only then in the material. Remember that dreams take time to realise. So too does the Law of Attraction.

CHAPTER 8

What about Luck or is it Something Else?

Have you ever looked at some people who just seem to have it all and asked yourself what makes them special? Do they have more angels on their side? How come they are so lucky?

In 2004 an English Professor, Richard Wiseman, published a book, *The Luck Factor*, which drew on the results of several years' research examining the behaviour, attitudes and experiences of hundreds of lucky and unlucky people.[118] His research identified that luck was not a birthright, nor did it somehow just happen to those who were classified lucky; rather, their luck essentially hinged on four principles.

So, what are these four principles? In summary they are:

- Principle 1 – Lucky people create, notice and act upon the chance opportunities of life (they are aware).

---

[118] Wiseman, R. 2004 *The Luck Factor* Arrow Books Great Britain

- Principle 2 – Lucky people listen to lucky hunches. They listen to their intuition.
- Principle 3 – Lucky people expect good fortune (you might call this visualisation.)
- Principle 4 – Lucky people seek to turn bad luck into good luck.

Through large experiments he also determined that luck was not a matter of psychic ability (did that person somehow know the winning lottery numbers?), nor was it a matter of intelligence, of conscientiousness or hard work. Rather, it was attitude that led people to be open to possibility.

It is important here to stop for a moment and reflect on what it means *to be open*. Does this mean that we just lie on the grass and wait for a possibility to happen? Or do our lives, thinking, language and conversations all reflect *the activity* of being open? Think of it in terms of being open to a new relationship. The way we approach, speak, and respond to members of the opposite sex will reflect an activity of being open, if only at a subconscious level.

If we look at Professor Wiseman's lucky people, we find that they lived out the expectations of their hearts. In the first principle listed above, consider all the activity words: *create*, *notice* and *act upon*. These people are consciously living life, hence again the importance of observation and of awareness.

If you seek, you will find, as the Bible puts it. If you visualise your dream, then as you begin to attract to yourself the makings of it, you will, at some level, notice those makings and act on them.

So, for instance, being open meant that these lucky people tended to network and socialise. They listened to their intuition; they were also open to the universe, rather than tending to notice only those things that were important to them at the moment whilst ignoring whatever else was in their surroundings, not least the opportunities.

Lucky people were found to be more relaxed; they would tend to *listen* to people, rather than seek to dominate a conversation. How many people even know how to listen? They then became aware of what there was to be seen in their world, rather than what they thought ought to be seen. They were not confined by the lens of their paradigms.

What happens in many conversations, not just with strangers and acquaintances, but also friends, is that we are so keen to tell them what we have to say that we only half listen, if at all, to the other person's dialogue. We have this desperate need to be noticed and heard, rather than to notice and to hear.

If so, we can miss the cues:

- that could tell us of new possibilities, of new directions;
- that might open our paradigms up and introduce us to whole new worlds; and
- maybe we also miss the cues because we, consciously or unconsciously, close off because of the other person's voice, clothes, or background and so miss those angelic messengers who would speak into our future through the medium of that person.

Stop here for a minute and ask yourself: Do I over-talk other people? Do I really listen? Do I select my conversational partners because of how they look, or sound, or their occupation or lack of it?

As we have noted throughout, being relaxed in ourselves is a part of this whole approach to life, this openness. Too often we engage in a social or work situation with an end game in mind. We focus on meeting the right people, saying the right thing, having a good time; or just plain focused on finding a partner, making an impression, clinching a deal, or reaching a destination, etcetera.

> **Do we focus on the visible *bars* that mark the boundary of our momentary existence? Are we blind to the *stars* that beckon us beyond, to the life-changing opportunities that are on offer?**

In so doing we focus on the *bars* that mark the boundary of our momentary existence and are blind to the *stars* that beckon us beyond, to the life-changing opportunities that are on offer.

In related fashion, Professor Wiseman notes that 'lucky people are open to new experiences in their lives.'[119] This is demanding. First and foremost, this challenges the self-imposed limits of our own world. It places an imperative on us to step outside what we know or had planned. It challenges our comfort zone – sometimes seriously so.

Secondly, lucky people expect the new experience to be positive. They have an outlook that expects the best, rather than believing in failure and disappointment as a normalcy.

How do we move to become a person with a sunny and open outlook on life; one who is prepared to grasp new experiences with high expectation? The answer is to start small. For instance, do you travel the same route to work every day, or follow a set routine? Do you live habitually? Just for once why don't you change it - mess with your mind and live dangerously! Do you find yourself always mixing with or talking to the same people? Break out and force yourself

---

[119] Wiseman, R. 2004 *The Luck Factor* Arrow Books Great Britain p57

to also begin mixing with new groups. You don't have to discard the old friends. Join a salsa dance class, as one friend of mine did; or a slow-cooking group, as another did. Simply speaking: broaden your world.

Meeting people from other cultures and from different backgrounds are recommended strategies to changing our thinking and so remove cognitive barriers that shape our paradigms, as previously outlined in Chapter Two.

My wife and I have had some of the richest moments of our lives when we have connected with people from radically different backgrounds, by joining or being involved with different interest groups.

Another factor is that of intuition – the hunch – the gut-feel, in a given situation, which we briefly looked at when we considered synchronicity.

Intuition is an interesting phenomenon. Literally, it is defined as '*instinctive knowing without the use of rational processes.*'[120] For some, and I believe that this is true, it is an aspect of the divine, or at least of the spirit life, of a person. As an unseen, unreasoned, process it is also a highly creative process.

'Listening to your intuition is the essence of art and creativity and soulful living. Intuition is what you use to find the purpose of your life and your place in the world. In philosophy, intuition is the power of obtaining knowledge that cannot be acquired either by inference or observation, by reason or experience.

---

[120] WordNet Retrieved 13 September 2007 from http://wordnet.princeton.edu/perl/webwn?s=intuition

As such, intuition is thought of as an original, independent source of knowledge, since it is designed to account for just those kinds of knowledge that other sources do not provide.' [121]

How do we cultivate it? Lucky people in Professor Wiseman's study not only listened to their intuition, but their intuition was strengthened by practicing stillness exercises, such as meditation, which relaxed their being, allowing them to hear from the small inner voice (notice that word *relax* again)

Lucky people also tended to clear their mind, find quiet places, and return to problems later. They allowed space and time to find the road through a situation or to the next staging post in life. As Elisabeth Kubler Ross once said, *'there is no need to go to India or anywhere else to find peace. You will find that deep place of silence right in your room, your garden or even your bathtub.'*

As discussed, relaxation and meditation are an integral part of the journey of the lucky person. We will return to this later in the book. It is so important.

I would also encourage you to read *The Luck Factor* which demonstrates scientifically the reality that luck is essentially a matter of an attitude towards life.

Professor Wiseman's research clearly revealed not only the opportunistic nature of the lucky individuals who participated, but also how they had lucky events occur that were clearly outside of their control, yet somehow, they were the beneficiaries of the WOW factor. The factor that causes those around them to scratch their heads in bemusement

---

[121] Angelfire. Retrieved 13 September 2007 from http://www.angelfire.com/hi/TheSeer/intuition.html

and say 'wow, the lucky devils, how come everything goes their way?' I am writing this to say that their experience is yours for the living if you really want it.

You too can be *lucky*.

CHAPTER 9

You, Your Brain and Your Thoughts

Changing our mind - the brain is plastic

FOR MANY CENTURIES THE BRAIN has been seen to be malleable during our childhood years, progressively becoming hard wired and then unchangeable as we reach the age of twenty. This concept 'grew out of, and was supported by, an Industrial Age metaphor that represented the brain as a mechanical contraption.'[122] This mechanical conclusion met all the requirements of Newtonian scientific rationalist thinking. Such thinking, as was outlined when the effect of paradigms was discussed, removed the possibilities for change and upward transformation in our lives.

---

[122] Carr, N., *The Shallows,* Atlantic Books, 2010 p1

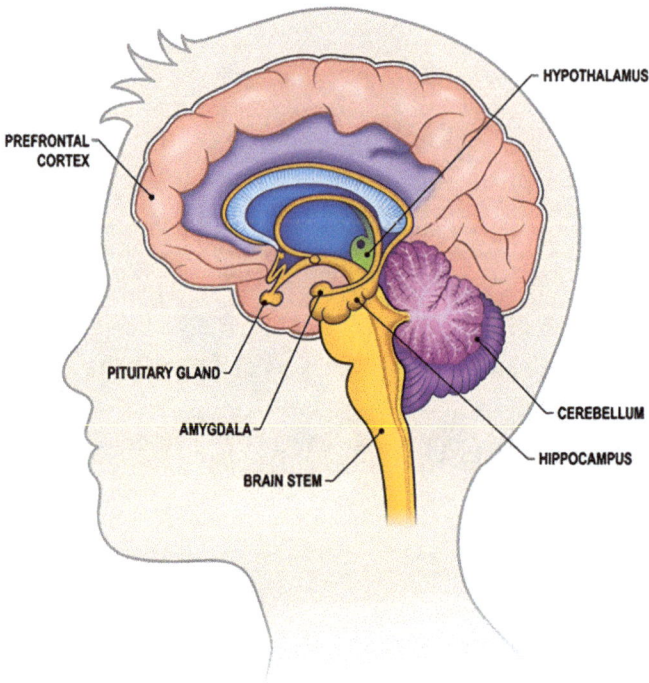

Figure 9.1: The human brain

> **"We never use the same brain twice".**
> Source: Research Perspectives of the Max Planck Society

Yet in an earlier chapter, we said the vehicle on our life's journey is our mind. This is only possible because our brains are not hard wired; they are plastic. They are changeable and can change not only in function, but in structure, through the activity of thinking. The activity of thinking changes both what we can do and the reality of our lives.

This is not science fiction, but established scientific fact, popularised by Norman Doidge, a research psychiatrist at Columbia University in his book *The Brain that Changes Itself*. The research behind the book stretches back for a number of decades and is now universally acknowledged in relevant scientific circles throughout the world.

Michael Greenberg, rather more poetically, wrote:

'The neurosystem in which this cascade of memory occurs, with its branches and transmitters and ingeniously spanned gaps, has an improvised quality that seems to mirror the unpredictability of thought itself. It is an ephemeral place that changes as our experience changes, to the point where we are incapable of remembering the same event in exactly the same way twice.'[123]

'The brain is a river not a rock'
(Fred Travis PhD.)

Contrary to popular belief, the brain's ability to change continues into old age. Dr Michael Merzenich writes that:

'Often, people think of childhood and young adulthood as a time of brain growth – the young person constantly learns new things, embarks on new adventures, (and) shows an inquisitive and explorative spirit. Conversely, older adulthood is often seen as a time of brain decline, with people becoming more forgetful, less inclined to seek new experiences, more "set in their ways". But what recent research has shown is that under the right circumstances the older brain can grow, too. Although certain brain machinery tends to decline with age, there are steps people can take to tap into plasticity and reinvigorate that machinery. We just have to "exercise" the brain in the right way'.[124]

One of the established keys to changing our lives is through the process of thinking differently or using thought processes in unusual ways. For instance, believe it or not, while not a substitute for physical training,

---

[123] Greenberg, M., 'Just remember this', New York Review of Books, December 2008

[124] Merzenich, M. 'About Brain Plasticity' Retrieved 27 December 2009 from http://merzenich.positscience.com/about-brain-plasticity/

imagined muscle movements increase muscle strength; visualised activities translate into enhanced performance.[125] These are practices known to, and adopted by, coaches around the world.

So, engaging in certain mental activities, including mindfulness meditation, cognitive training programs, and even simply focusing on positive thoughts, has been shown to lead to changes in brain structure and function. These changes can positively impact things like attention, memory, emotional regulation, and even cognitive reserve, which can protect against neurodegenerative diseases.

Brain cells that fire together stay together

Thoughts lead to the creation of new synapses in the brain. And as we shall see, changing what is possible.

The brain is the engine room of our thoughts. It is the operating hardware behind our soul on which our thinking programs run. As it is so central to our lives and our well-being, an understanding of the human brain, how it works, and how it is best supported by us, will pay big dividends.

In the space of a single chapter, I would not pretend to canvass all the intricacies of the brain, but rather endeavour to highlight some aspects that affect the way we can actualise our potential.

Our brain is the most complicated organism on the planet with over 100 billion nerve cells and more connections than there are stars in the sky. Information in the brain travels at 431 kilometres (or 268 miles) per hour. On average, 85,000 brain cells die per day. Brain cells are unusual in their own right. For example, the cells don't link

---

[125] Research from the Cleveland Clinic Foundation in Ohio

148

up permanently. Reflect for a second – this is different to how your body cells connect, isn't it?

But brain cells would not be much good if they never connected at all. In fact, as soon as you are born, they make connections according to your life experience. These connections between neurons, or their tentacle branches known as dendrites, are called synapses. The synapse is a tiny space because the neurons don't actually touch. This is the synaptic gap.

The brain cells send electrical/chemical messengers across the space of the synapses. These messengers act like couriers with packets of information. The pathways that are formed by this activity are created, grow or diminish, and ultimately disappear according to how much the neural connection is used. For example, if you play the piano, then the relevant connections in the brain grow and strengthen, but if you give it up, then these connections become weaker and eventually will fall away. That is to say:

'Brain cells that fire together stay together.'[126]

In the early years of life there is a nearly blank cognitive slate which is waiting to be written on. For while brain development is protected during pregnancy by the general health and well-being of the mother, the first two years of life heralds the period of the most rapid brain organisation.

'A baby's brain is dynamically developing from birth with most of the essential neuronal connections established by the age of three, enabling the child to regulate emotions, communicate, solve problems, and form relationships.'[127]

---

[126] Hebbs law summarised by Carla Shatz

[127] Submission No. 13 from National Investment for The Early Years, p1.

Brain organisation precedes function. This is important at all stages of our lives. For example, *'we know from brain neurological connection time, the key time for the neuronal connection for readiness for literacy is about the six-month mark.'*[128] This is the more remarkable as a child at six months cannot even speak yet. It highlights the importance of patience and preparation. It is why it is important to read to the infant at this age and doing so is a metaphor for the Law of Attraction since it anticipates a believed future outside of the presenting reality.

What we allow our brain to think about is the single most powerful factor in creating who we are! This is because our thinking (our mind) actually and demonstrably creates the pathways in our brain. The act of thinking and how we respond is what makes our brains plastic. The more we travel a particular road, the more lit up, or stimulated, our brain cells become. As our brain changes, so to do our perceptions. There is a virtuous circle of improvement. Remember this when we look at the practical exercises towards the end of this book.

Reality is interpreted perception

Because our perceptions can change, we need to hold them lightly. Consider this: perceptions are not reality itself. They may be pretty good approximations, but they are never complete and entirely true. For example, consider going for a walk with a dog – the dog hears ultrasonic noises and smells things you do not, but you see in colour (presumably) while the dog does not. Physical reality is the same for both of you, but your perception, and thus your experience of it, will be different. Nor is reality the same for the brain injured. Head injuries, strokes, attention-deficit/hyperactivity disorder (ADHD), depression, and so on all predispose people to be selective in what they notice about reality,

---

[128] Dr Trevor Parry, *National Investment for the Early Years (WA), Transcript of Evidence*, 25 March 2009, p4.

or particularly distortive. Reality is interpreted perception. Classically, eyewitness accounts can be influenced by factors such as stress, fear, and personal biases, leading to inaccurate recollections of events.

What we think about is formed largely by desire, and desire is the prism that focuses our thinking, allowing it to become transformatory. This can work to both our benefit and our detriment. Advantageously, visualising or thinking about playing a particular piece of music or practicing a golf swing or running a race has been shown repeatedly to enhance performance. Detrimentally, for example, pornography, driven by sexual desire, can both shape and pervert our sexual behaviour as it moulds the plasticity of our brain through the activation of the brain's pleasure centres.

> **Our life, our thinking, changes because there is a desire that shapes a commitment that determines an action.**

This demonstrates a reality. Lives do not get changed just because we feel it would be nice to be different or live differently. Our life, our thinking, changes because there is a desire that shapes a commitment that determines an action.

The brain is divided into different sections that perform different jobs. Its structure, however, is far more flexible than once thought. If one part fails, then it is sometimes possible for other parts to take over the function of the failed part. For example, recent research has demonstrated that a surprising number of stroke victims who have not responded to traditional therapeutic interventions can be taught to respond through such brain altering interventions as Constraint Induced Movement Therapy[129] which rewires the brain's circuitry.

---

[129] After a stroke, constraint-induced movement therapy (CI) forces the use of the affected side of the body by restraining the unaffected side. For example, with CI therapy, the therapist constrains the survivor's unaffected arm in a sling. The survivor then uses his or her affected arm repetitively and intensively for two weeks

Such interventions have also proven beneficial to children affected by cerebral palsy, providing further evidence for the plasticity of the brain. Subsequent changes in function within the brain can be readily evidenced through brain scans. In very general terms, all areas of the brain adapt to a change in any one area of the brain because of the wealth of neurological connections to and from each area. What this means is that we have far greater potential capacity in our brain than we are ever likely to use. One reason we do not use that capacity is the pre-existing paradigm that limits our belief as to what is possible, as was the case with the treatment of stroke victims before Constraint Induced Movement Therapy.

In creating consciously, we learn to use both the left and right brains, and life gets much easier. We all would want that! Our brains can be used in a helpful, holistic way or they can be used in a partial, unbalanced, or fragmented way. Since we are habitual, we use our brains in an unbalanced and fragmented way. This is because habitual behaviour creates mental tracks in our brain's circuitry which we will unthinkingly follow. Seeking to use the whole mind is important because the quality of your entire life can be transformed if you change your brain functioning. Many of life's illusions, difficulties, and limitations can then be addressed.

Looking after your brain:

The brain is that part of our being which allows us to recognise our own humanity – '*I think, therefore I am.*' [130] It is the seat of our cognition and of our emotions. It is the source of our imagination and, perhaps, the locus of our soul. It can help us create the reality we choose and

---

[130] René Descartes, a French philosopher, summarised his position in this famous quote.

define the boundaries of our existence. This being so, how we look after it should be very important.

Looking after the brain is not simply about maintenance, it is also about enhancement. Nowhere is this truer than for those of us who are sufferers of mental afflictions. Anxiety is one of the more common of those afflictions. The definition of anxiety is fear in the absence of immediate threat. We can suffer because mental disturbances, such as depression or anxiety, can create their own long-lasting pathways on our plastic neural circuitry that reinforce the condition. Anxiety, in particular, can become a lasting condition that steadily gets worse with age, contributing to depression. It takes a conscious effort to recreate the direction of those pathways but change them we can.

Since the brain is plastic, we can change its functioning; and we can change our lives. We can change our lives because our brain is an intrinsic part of our being that defines the reality of our existence through the electric signals it receives through the five senses. Reality is interpreted perception, and the brain is the window to our reality.

Dr Daniel Amen[131], in a lecture recorded on the Internet, speaks at length on the brain (http://amenclinics.com/server1). Dr Amen argues, like many others, that because of its very plasticity, you can change the way the brain serves you.

His key principles relative to the brain may be summarised as follows:

   i)   Your brain is involved in everything you do. Your brain
        is involved in what you think (and thoughts change your
        reality), how you act, and how you get along with people. It

---

[131] A Distinguished Fellow of the American Psychiatric Association and, amongst other things, the CEO and Medical Director of Amen Clinics, Inc.

is the organiser of your personality, your intelligence, and is the hardware of your soul.

ii) When the brain works right, then you work right. When the brain is in trouble, then so are you.

iii) Your brain is as soft as butter with a consistency not much different to custard and, whilst encased in a very hard skull, – it is vulnerable.

iv) You can change your brain, and so your thoughts and beliefs.

v) Many things can help your brain function better or diminish its functionality.

First, positively, you can help your brain with:

i) Anything that increases blood flow helps, such as exercise.

ii) Meditation, which appears in a later chapter of this book, activates the most thoughtful part of the brain. It improves both our mood and our memory and enables us to make better decisions.

iii) Ensuring you get enough sleep.

iv) Constant learning and socialising. New learning creates new connections in our brain.

v) Having an attitude of gratitude – this creates a positive outlook which enhances brain function in trying situations. The functional brain scan of a thankful person reflects the fact that the whole mind is switched on – conscious and unconscious. Just by the attitude of gratitude we recondition the body. What is more significant is that you can give thanks for what we have not received yet. This signals the body, which knows no better, that it has happened already and when the mind and the body are on the same page, we have the power of the universe behind us.

vi) A good brain diet, which includes:
   • Plenty of water.

- Omega-3 rich food such as avocado, fish oil, salmon, tuna and walnuts.
- Antioxidants, such as green tea and blueberries.
- Vitamin C as you might find in oranges or red bell peppers, for example.

Second, on the negative side, the following will hurt your brain's functionality:

i) Drugs, including excessive alcohol.
ii) High levels of bad stress – lack of stress management leads to reduced blood flow to the brain.
iii) Toxic fumes.
iv) Excess caffeine – Dr Amen suggests that two cups of coffee a day is an elegant sufficiency, so to speak.
v) Cigarettes, as these work to reduce the blood flow to your brain.
vi) Less than six hours sleep a night (for most people) will reduce the blood flow to the brain.

Notice how much Dr Amen's findings overlap and are congruent with Professor Wiseman's findings on so called lucky people.

The question to ask yourself is this: *Is my behaviour, day in and day out, helping or hurting my brain?*

The tripartite nature of our brain

Our brain, for our purposes here, comprises three sections:

- the pre-frontal cortex;
- the cingulated gyrus; and
- the limbic system.

It is important to understand the role and effect of these areas of the brain as they affect our behaviour and make us what we are as individuals and as a species.

The pre-frontal cortex – free will

This area of the brain is thought to be involved in planning and complex cognitive behaviours and in the expression of personality and appropriate social behaviour.[132] What separates us from all other sentient species is that the frontal lobe of our brain is the most developed. This is what makes us human and differentiates us from other animal species. It forms at least 30% of the human brain (compared to 11% in chimpanzees and 7% in dogs). This is the location of the executive functions of the brain. This is where we exercise forethought, control, judgement, empathy, and learning from experience.

This is the place where free will is located. Where there is a *free will*, then please understand that there is also a *free won't*; that is to say that we also have the ability to say no. The frontal lobe is, in fact, also the place where the free won't is located; that executive inhibitor of response that stops us from running amok.

When there are problems here, we see patterns of procrastination. Bad judgement and a lack of learning from experiences are all evident. Some symptoms include a lack of focus, low energy, and a need for a crisis to work properly.

Crisis, or the sense of crisis and even conflict, stimulates activity in the brain. Have you ever worked with people who only seem to thrive

---

[132] Brain explorer Retrieved 23 March 2008 from http://www.brainexplorer.org/glossary/prefrontal_cortex.shtml

when there is a crisis? Dr Amen suggests that the treatment for these problems include:

- writing goals for all areas of your life and repeating them daily;
- daily exercise;
- high protein and low carbohydrate diet (only if this is your area of difficulty); and
- fish oil.

So, if this is where your free will is located, then what is free will? It is the ability to consciously make a choice. In choosing, you are always selecting a future. Your future is not pre-determined as we have seen. We do not live in a Newtonian mechanical universe. Free will and Quantum Physics resonate with each other as we live in a sea of possibility and probability, creating multiple futures, each carrying their different possibilities.

What does this have to do with us and the Law of Attraction?

We know we can use our pre-frontal cortex in mental rehearsing or visualisation to enhance performance as it is successfully used by coaches and athletes. It is also used by actors and concert pianists. Mental rehearsing helps the mind, or imagination, 'make it so'. Brain scans show that imagining an activity and doing it are not that different, which is why this works. This demonstrable fact, which is replicated every day the world over, can be used to your great advantage.

In an interview in the film *What the Bleep*, Dr. Joe Dispenza illustrates this with a personal example:

'I wake up in the morning and I consciously create my day the way I want it to happen. Now sometimes, because my mind is

examining all the things that I need to get done, it takes me a little bit to settle down and get to the point of where I'm actually intentionally creating my day. But here's the thing: When I create my day and out of nowhere little things happen that are so unexplainable, I know that they are the process or the result of my creation. And the more I do that, the more I build a neural net in my brain that I accept that that's possible. [This] gives me the power and the incentive to do it the next day.' [133]

Situationally, not only is performance enhanced through the process of mentally creating the day, but the subsequent events of the day then have a quantum-like predisposition to draw into themselves the necessary ingredients to facilitate the envisaged outcome.

Unfortunately, most people only partially use the frontal lobe and so could be said to be operating with a *frontal lobe lobotomy*, choosing to respond to situations habitually and with habitual behaviour. Because what we think we know is always going to be limited, we tend to get stuck on how to change our thinking. We also prefer habitual thinking to the effort of creating our day. We have a vague *what will be, will be* approach that, while not making us victims, certainly makes us inattentive to our attitudinal address to life. This may be so because we do not believe how we think about things is going to make much of a difference anyway... How wrong we are!

---

[133] What the bleep Retrieved 20 November 2007 from http://www.whatthebleep.com/create/

The cingulated gyrus – the gear shifter of the brain[134]

The second part of the brain we should look at is the cingulated gyrus. This part has three key functions:

- it coordinates sensory input with emotions;
- it provides our emotional responses to pain; and
- it regulates aggressive behaviour.[135]

As Doctor Amen[136] puts it, this part of our brain is the gear shifter of our mind. It allows us to shift our attention, to be flexible, and to see options and is involved in error detection. Problems in this part of the brain often arise through a lack of serotonin and then people can get stuck in obsessions, holding grudges, and becoming inflexible – their gear has stuck.

Dr Amen suggests that the best way to respond to any problems here is:

- if there is a thought that comes into your head more than three times then you need to distract yourself and get up and go for a walk;
- if someone else is stuck – give them options, not a single direction; and
- use reverse psychology on them, tell the person to do the opposite of what you want them to do. The classic example is one which many parents have used when a pre-schooler threatens to leave home and the parent offers to help them pack.

---

[134] 'Change Your Brain, Change Your Life.' Retrieved 23 March 2008 from http://amenclinics.com/server1

[135] About.com Biology Retrieved 23 March 2008 from http://biology.about.com/library/organs/brain/blcingyrus.htm

[136] 'Change Your Brain, Change Your Life.' Retrieved 23 March 2008 from http://amenclinics.com/server1

The limbic – the emotional brain – the seat of reaction

The limbic system is sometimes referred to as the emotional brain. In evolutionary terms it is the oldest part of the brain.

> *'The limbic is not a single organ but a cluster of distinct organs, each with specific and diverse functions. The three organs that generate and control our emotions — the thalamus, hypothalamus, and the amygdala — are part of the region and aggregate of organs we call the limbic brain.*[137]

The limbic system maintains the balance in our lives, controlling temperature, how thirsty we feel, how hungry we feel, our hormonal flows, and equilibrium. It is the central computer which runs below our consciousness. It sets our emotional tone; it drives us to love, to joy, and how positive or negative we feel. It may be said to be the seat of our pleasure centres. This is where dopamine works on our brain. For instance, falling in love triggers the threshold of this area of the brain making us sensitive to the things around us that might be pleasurable. In opening us up it rewires our plastic brain, creating neurological links of association. Who has not smelled a scent, or seen a face that has not thrown us back by association to a place or a time? This is the part of the brain where it happens. Emotions are the greatest rewirers of our mind and, when we are passionate about wanting something, our emotion-laden thoughts cause things to happen. The impossible becomes attainable.

The limbic system is involved with our ability to connect to others. It processes our sense of smell and manages our libido.

---

[137] Project Renaissance Retrieved 23 March 2008 from http://www.winwenger.com/limbic1.htm

The Amygdala

Inside the limbic system is the amygdala. This almond-shaped structure stores the emotional perceptions that occur each time memory is built. Every time we build or relive a memory, we activate the emotions associated with that memory. In doing so, we can further reinforce the previously established neurological pathways that dictate patterns in our behaviour.

> **Even when the stressors have disappeared, the amygdala can remain enlarged, leading to sustained or chronic anxiety and heightened reactivity.**

A problem arises for us when the emotions activated are those stored from our early years when rationality was not strong. Such emotionally charged moments, raw and reactive, can flood our system in later life, triggering responses that another part of us can recognise as being over the top, or unreasonable.

At an everyday level we will often make mountains out of molehills and perceive stressors that don't even exist, except in our imagination, that is. This ramps up our stress levels and our anxiety and takes a toll on our mental and physical health. The results of worrying about what has not happened is the main reason there are more heart attacks on Monday mornings prior to work than at any other time in the week.[138]

Such over-activation of the stress response in our daily lives has a number of lasting effects on our physiology, as well as our psychology. To name just two:

---

[138] Dr Craig Hassed MBBS, FRACGP, *The health benefits of meditation and being mindful, Available at: http://www.49.com.au/wp-content/uploads/The-health-benefits-of-meditation-and-being-mindful_v21-2.pdf*

- loss of brain cells (accelerated ageing or atrophy), particularly in the hippocampus and prefrontal cortex (learning, memory and executive functioning areas of the brain), which predisposes to Alzheimer's Disease in later life; and
- growth of the amygdala (the fear and stress centre of the brain).

The growth of the amygdala is significant, as it creates a perpetually heightened sense of fight or flight readiness in us. This 'overactive stress centre (amygdala) 'highjack's' this area of the brain making normal functioning effectively difficult if not impossible.[139] Even when the stressors have disappeared, research shows that the amygdala can remain enlarged, leading to sustained or chronic anxiety and a heightened sense of reactivity.

Memory and emotions are inseparable. In a normal brain, the amygdala acts as an early warning system, triggering fears and reactions to those fears unconsciously which might have saved our hunter-gatherer forebears' lives millennia ago, but are often redundant in our daily lives today.

Taking the brain as a whole, the limbic system running below our consciousness is, I would suggest, the seat of the 'moving centre'[140] of our behaviour and is the enabler of habitual living.

---

[139] ibid

[140] *The moving center* is that part of our being that regulates our behavior and responses at an unconscious level. These behaviors may have arisen through repeated experience or learning or may be innate, such as our fight or flight response to perceived threats.

Habitual living happens because the neural networks linked to habits of thinking and behaviour are like a path through the woods. The more you walk a path the more established it becomes.[141]

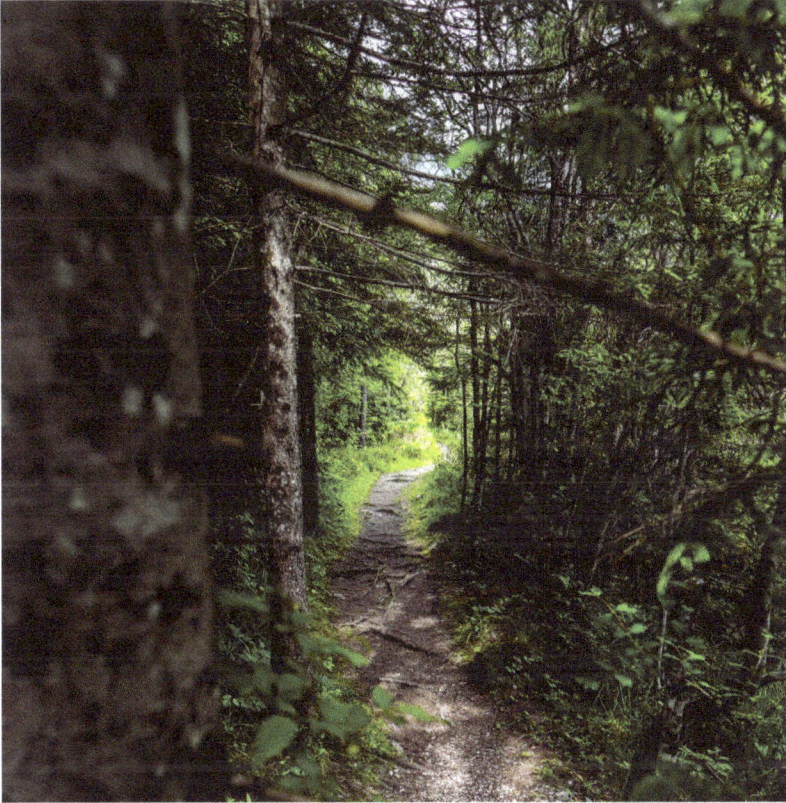

The more your mind and body travels the same path, the stronger those connections become ingrained and so many behaviours become unthinking.

Just as behaviours become unthinking, so too may our responses to our environment. When there are problems here, you might feel

---

[141] Bergland, C. 'The Athletes Way' Available: https://www.psychologytoday. com/blog/the-athletes-way/201311/the-size-and-connectivity-the-amygdala-pre- dicts-anxiety

depressed, helpless, hopeless, or sad, wracked with guilt or simply have a lot of negative thoughts running through your day and you are not quite sure why.

Remember, this is a background computer program and what it is feeding you is not necessarily understood, only experienced.

> **After an eight week course in Mindfulness meditation, the amygdala, associated with fear and emotion, shrinks while the prefrontal cortex, associated with awareness, concentration and decision making, grows thicker.**
> Dr Joe Dispenza

It is recognised that one of the values of psychotherapy is that it improves the ability of our pre-frontal cortex, that seat of free will, to regulate the behaviour of the limbic system. When emotions are unregulated by your prefrontal cortex, then the civilised part of our nature is overruled through the amygdala. We can flare up in a way that can cause us subsequent embarrassment.

When we behave in this way, we want to isolate ourselves. Have you ever yelled at a driver of another car for doing something that seemed careless, and then realised it was someone you knew? Perhaps you have let your anger explode in a relationship, whether it's with your children, a colleague or a partner and so begun a slow corrosive process in the relationship.

The answer is to be aware of your emotions and your reactions in different situations. We have in ourselves the ability to trigger a relaxation response, which is opposite to the stress response.

Count to ten before responding. In neurobiological terms – extend the authority of your prefrontal cortex over the limbic/amygdala.

This is best achieved through the scientifically researched practice of Mindfulness, which we will look at later in this book.

Some benefits of Mindfulness-based meditation are the generation of new brain cells (neurogenesis), particularly in the memory and executive functioning centres, dementia prevention, and reduced activity in the amygdala.

Mindfulness practice through our awareness gives us space in which to choose rationally how to respond to reactive situations.

When we are depressed, angry or anxious, we can stand back and try reframing the situation in which we find ourselves. We can try to see it differently – and ask how someone else would view it.

Besides Mindfulness, other strategies that give our prefrontal cortex greater opportunity to gain control over the limbic system when it seems to be running amok are:

- Regularly maintained exercise. This lowers our adrenalin and improves the oxygen level in our bloodstream and to our brain. It is also self-discipline. Without adrenalin, the heat of our anger dissipates rapidly.
- Fish oil supplements – many depressed people are found to be deficient in this nutrient and people in countries with high fish diets have the lowest rates of depression.

The Brain – who is in charge?

So, you have decided to look after your brain now that you are aware of its needs, and you are a bit clearer as to how this marvel works for you: what is next?

In terms of the brain, how do we make sense of the world we live in? How do we change the world we live in? These two questions are closely intertwined, as are the answers to them.

The brain is a pathway to, and helps form, our higher self. The brain is not only changed through evolutionary processes and not only by inherited genetic mutation, although both of these are true to differing degrees. As discussed, because the brain is plastic, each individual's brain develops an individual biological structure as the networks of the brain adapt, connect, or disconnect according to the activities and thought processes of that individual.

Both the quantity and the quality of neurological networks can be enhanced through our thoughts and activities, forming new modules of functionality. In fact, the very structure of the brain is demonstrably changeable; however, it is the repetition of thoughts and actions that form new modules of functionality.

The brain contains what some would refer to as the essence of our being and of our consciousness, our soul, if you like. Because it runs on electro chemical signals it is also that part of us that is closest to the universe, that medium and facilitator of life and to God/Creator, the unseen source and inspiration for our lives.

Strengthening our connection to the higher self[142] can radically shift our energy and life on all levels of being. *'It allows us to see through the veils of illusion, misperceptions and faulty beliefs to the true nature of reality, the truth of who we are and the love at the heart of our being.'*[143] And it all starts with our thinking. This is not always an easy process.

---

[142] Our 'spiritual' being as opposed to our physical being
[143] Email from Aine Belton, 24 March 2008 of www.beliefbusterkit.com.

Every result in life starts as a thought, but our thoughts, constrained as they are by what we know and by our paradigms, can also be our blinkers. Unsurprisingly, as we age, it becomes harder and harder to make the necessary effort to break free from established patterns and ways of thinking. Therefore, as we get older, we try to preserve the familiar.

We become more conservative in our thinking and behaviour and, rather than change our internal neuro cognitive structures, we try and change the world around us to better suit our imagined reality.

We micromanage our environment, rather than confront the need to think and, therefore, to behave differently.[144] For example, we may choose like-minded friends, or we make travel arrangements that fall within our established comfort zone.

Even more significantly, as we have seen the limbic system stimulates our emotions, through chemicals such as adrenalin and serotonin, which impact our thinking. Many would argue that in reality we think by feeling.

This may sound bizarre but if there was a total lack of emotion would you care enough to respond to life's situations, what food you ate, what clothes you wore, what someone might think of you, and so on? Indeed:

> *'Where the study of emotion was once relegated to the backwaters of neuroscience, a testament to the popular conception that what we feel exists outside our brains, acting only to intrude on normal thought, the science has changed. Emotion is now considered integral*

[144] Doidge, N. 2007, *The Brain that changes itself,* Scribe Publications, Melbourne p305

to our over-all mental health. In mapping our emotions, scientists have found that our emotional brain overlays our thinking brain.'[145]

In ground-breaking research in the early 1970s, Amos Tversky and Daniel Kahnemann published their findings in relation to the way our rational mind is overridden by the limbic system. Kahnemann was subsequently awarded a Nobel Prize for his work. They found that even when logic told people what was correct, the limbic system could trump the pre-frontal cortex with an emotion-based response. One only has to think of the way romantic love or lust can make a fool of the most rational of us, sometimes even destroying careers and pre-existing relationships, to recognise the truth of this.

Our emotional brain overlays our thinking brain.

In another example, post-9/11 aircraft ticket sales slumped and took twelve months to recover. Logically, it was statistically highly unlikely that another event of that nature would occur so soon. Not only that, statistically, by resorting to driving, an individual's chance of death rose, as the likelihood of a fatal car accident is far higher than any aircraft disaster, intended or accidental. In fact, in that twelve-month period the death toll on roads rose comparably to the fall in airline ticket sales as more road trips were undertaken.

Given the way our limbic system influences us, at an unconscious level, we will fail to both recognise and take advantage of the possibilities life presents, as well as events that are outside of our patterned paradigm[146] of experience.

---

[145] The Secret Life of the brain, Retrieved 24 August 2009 from http://www.pbs. org/wnet/brain/episode4/index.html

[146] As mentioned - A paradigm may be defined as a set of assumptions, concepts, values, and practices that constitutes the way we view reality

The fact is that we believe we are logical; that the world in which we live can be seen and understood from where we are sitting; and that if we search, we will find, provided that we know what we are looking for. This is not, however, the whole story. We can only be logical at a conscious or cognitive level.

The larger part of the story is that, for a good reason, much of our lives are lived at an unconscious level, from the practice of breathing, to finding our way home. The unconscious mind is where habitual behaviour exists. Once you have learned to ride a bicycle without falling off the instinctual corrective behaviours reside in your unconscious. Your conscious mind may take control when you need to deal with the unexpected or make key decisions, perhaps how to handle a particular traffic situation. Even then, those responses may come from an unconscious assessment of the situation based on experience. Indeed, even when we are conscious and seemingly focussed, we can be blind-sided by our expectations. For instance, we do not expect cars to drive through red lights, but sometimes they do!

An interesting experiment (http://viscog.beckman.uiuc.edu/grafs/ demos/15.html) reveals how selective we are when we focus on a task. The video clip shows two teams of basketball players. The task is to count the number of times one team (white shirts) passes the ball to members of their own team. World-wide it has been found that if people are unaware that there is more to the video than that task, over 50% fail to notice a gorilla that walks across the court and stops in the middle of the players to beat his chest before moving off. The reason is simply that we are told to focus on the team of white shirts and the gorilla is in a black costume.

I was in a lecture room of some 100 people when this video clip was shown (with a suitable task-focusing preamble) and only two people saw the gorilla. Observers typically are shocked that they could have missed it. These videos, created by Daniel Simons and his students, show that when people focus their attention on a task or some aspect of life, they often fail to see unexpected objects and events.

There is a deep significance for all of us in this.

In our daily lives, we tend to be focussed on something or other, whether it's our emotions, a situation, or a task. This is especially true of men.[147]

Secondly, we may be blinded to what is around us by the way we think. This is because in our daily lives, our conscious thinking is based on pattern recognition and pattern matching intelligence, not information processing. We run what we see through the patterns in our long-term memories to see what matches. We have, in fact, evolved to quickly make decisions based on partial data recognition – on patterns. So, if you are faced with jumbled letters as follows you could probably still read it:

> *Aoccdrnig to a rscheearch at Cmabrigde Uinervtisy, it deosn't mttaer in waht oredr the ltteers in a wrod are, the olny iprmoetnt tihng is taht the frist and lsat ltteer be at the rghit pclae. The rset can be a toatl mses and you can sitll raed it wouthit porbelm. Tihs is bcuseae the huamn mnid deos not raed ervey lteter by istlef, but the wrod as a wlohe.*

And you probably could read it as follows:

> According to a researcher at Cambridge University, *'it doesn't matter in what order the letters in a word are, the only important*

---

[147] Research shows that men's and women's brains are fundamentally different, with one better at focusing, one better at multitasking.

thing is that the first and last letter be at the right place. The rest can be a total mess and you can still read it without a problem. This is because the human mind does not read every letter by itself but the word as a whole.[148]

It is the pattern which allows us to read the jumble, not the clarity of the information.

'Imagination is more important than knowledge.'
Albert Einstein

It seems that whatever we perceive is organised into patterns, for which we, the perceivers, are largely responsible… As perceivers, we select from all the stimuli falling on our senses only those which interest us, and our interests are governed by a pattern-making tendency, sometimes called a schema.

In a chaos of shifting impressions each of us constructs a stable world in which objects have recognisable shapes, are located in depth and have permanence. As times goes on and experience builds up, we make greater investment in our systems of labels. So a conservative bias is built in. It gives us confidence.[149]

I believe this move to a conservative bias, as we get older, is why children will sometimes see much more in the spiritual realm than adults do. Children are unimpeded in their thinking by historic schemas or patterns. As children, we also tend to be (clumsily) artistic in one form or another, often to a greater extent than we will as adults. This is probably because art and spirituality are far more free-floating

---

[148] Source: anonymous circular internet email

[149] Mary Douglas, Purity and Danger 1966 Retrieved 21 September 2007 from http://www.cognitive-edge.com/ceresources/presentations/9_2007_06_NDM_Monterey.pdf

aspects of the human soul. These aspects are in tune with the as yet unsorted chaos of shifting impressions, referred to above. While creativity is enhanced by learning, as we grow older, we become more affected by the views of others, and this inhibits our creativity.

This developing conservative bias will close us to those patterns outside of those that we expect to see. In other words, we will tend to see only what we are looking for. If you think by studying data you will see what you need to see, then you are likely to be mistaken. Rather, you will see what you expect to see in the light of your existing paradigms.

This is true as much at the very literal level of eyesight as it is in terms of discernment. In terms of our eyesight, the amazing thing is that the brain can compensate for certain visual aberrations without our even being aware of it.

'Retinal images in the human eye are affected by optical aberrations that cannot be corrected with ordinary spectacles or contact lenses, and the specific pattern of these aberrations is different in every eye. Though these aberrations always blur the retinal image, our subjective impression is that the visual world is sharp and clear, suggesting that the brain might compensate for their subjective influence.'[150]

With respect to discernment, however, when our brain interprets situations in the light of our held paradigms and beliefs, then such blinkered vision, at an extremity, can cost us our lives.

---

[150] Artal, P. et al., 'Neural compensation for the eye's optical aberrations', *Journal of Vision*, vol. 4, no.4, p281-287.

Philip Yancy[151] recounts how the poet and writer, John Donne, tells a story of a group of Spanish sailors who reached South America and sailed into the vast expanses of the headwaters of the Amazon which they simply assumed were an extension of the Atlantic Ocean. 'It never occurred to them to drink the water since *they expected* it to be saline, and as a result some of the sailors died of thirst.'

That scene of the sailors dying of thirst even as their ships floated on the world's largest source of fresh water is a metaphor for our age and our blindness. We can talk of the unseen worlds, of unseen spiritual truths, and the question is why are they unseen? Why are we blind to them?

Where do these patterns that frame the way we see our world come from? The answer is pretty straightforward.

- Our genetics
- Our life experience
- Our stories – think of the media, as well as the stories told to you by families, friends and work colleagues.

Between stimulus and response there is a space. In that space is our power to choose our response. In our response lies our growth and our freedom.

Unfortunately, whilst our experiences and stories could be positive or negative, we have evolved to pay more attention to the negative – it's all about survival.

In the normal course of events then, it becomes difficult for you, or me, to break out of our worldview or our paradigm and then innovate in the way that The IDEA is challenging you to do.

---

[151] Yancy, P. 1995 *Finding God in unexpected places* Hodder & Stoughton Great Britain p3

Our patterns are our interpretation of life and tell us who we are. They become our identity. The required changes in thinking become much easier when the patterns in our memory become temporarily unsustainable; for instance, when we are faced with starvation or a major life crisis of such a dimension that it disrupts the patterns, because they are not working for us in the moment.

None of us would wish to go to such dire extremes as fasting for 40 days and nights to force our minds to become open again; and indeed, for the most part it is unnecessary.

As recent science demonstrates, our brain remains malleable into old age, contrary to previous understanding. Because our brains are plastic, we can consciously change the functioning of the brain in ways that will enhance our lives. By using our prefrontal cortex, we can change pre-existing habits, paradigms and thinking patterns and so modify our responses to the situations we face in our daily lives. As Viktor Frankl, survivor of the holocaust wrote:

> *'Between stimulus and response there is a space. In that space is our power to choose our response. In our response lies our growth and our freedom.'*

CHAPTER 10

Taking Charge –
Managing our Brain Waves

CONSIDER FOR A MOMENT THE relationship of the brain to the Law of Attraction. To tap into the potential that the Law of Attraction would give us and our lives requires a break in our patterning, and it requires activity on our part. To achieve that break, we need to put ourselves in a particular mental state.

How do we do that? Think for a moment of the well-established fact that we can change our emotions and our health by changing the electronic wave pattern of our brains. Some of the research on this issue is considered when we discuss meditation later.

> **Brainwaves are the signature of what is going on inside of our minds.**
> Source: Brainwave College

We have seen that higher intelligence, through the engaged mind, controls and alters the brain's manner of functioning — that is, the brain is a function of human intelligence through the mind. We can also correlate brain wave frequencies with mind activity. Or we could put it another way – our state of mind can be determined by our brain waves and if we can change the frequency of our brain waves, we can change our state of mind. Brainwaves are actually the signature of what is going on inside of our minds.

What are brain waves and why do they matter?

Well, the dictionary definition of a brain wave is not a 'bright idea' as some would have it but, and I quote:

> 'Brainwaves (neurophysiology) are rapid fluctuations of voltage between parts of the cerebral cortex that are detectable with an electroencephalograph.'[152]

We saw earlier that the brain operates on chemical/electrical impulses. Brain waves are the fluctuations in those impulses, the frequency of which can be measured.

> 'A frequency is the number of times a wave repeats itself within a second. It can be compared to the frequencies that you tune into on your radio. If any of these frequencies are deficient, excessive, or difficult to access, our mental performance can suffer.'[153]

What is important in considering brainwaves is that not only do they reflect the activity of our brains but, if we control the frequency, we can change our mood, our thinking and even our behaviour; so, it is a two-way street. How does this happen?

---

[152] Princeton Retrieved 24 March 2008 from http://wordnet.princeton.edu/perl/webwn?s=brain%20wave

[153] Crossroads Institute Retrieved 24 March 2008 from http://www.crossroadsinstitute.org/eeg.html

The activity of our brains is based on our reactions to situations around us in our daily lives. The frequency of our brain waves will reflect our reactions. We can, however, use our brain waves to put ourselves in the best possible state of mind to deal with those situations, instead of simply reacting. We can control our minds and better master the situation facing us.

This is important because, as someone once asked: 'Is it the situation around you, or the way you react to the situation, that's causing the problem?'

In this context it is interesting to note, as expanded on below, that the frequency of our brain waves affects the release of such hormones as adrenalin, endorphins, and human growth hormones which are produced by the pituitary gland in the human brain.

Brain waves are an immensely exciting field of learning because they can give us such a significant level of control on our lives. Whole movements of learning have evolved to teach people how to radically change their lives through the understanding and control of their mind, not least their brain waves, for example, the Silva Mind Control Method.

The five main frequencies of brain waves in order of the level of their frequency, from high to low, are Gamma, Beta, Alpha, Theta, and Delta.

Of these, four are more popularly known and understood, namely Beta, Alpha, Theta and Delta.

The relative frequencies of these brain waves is illustrated as follows:

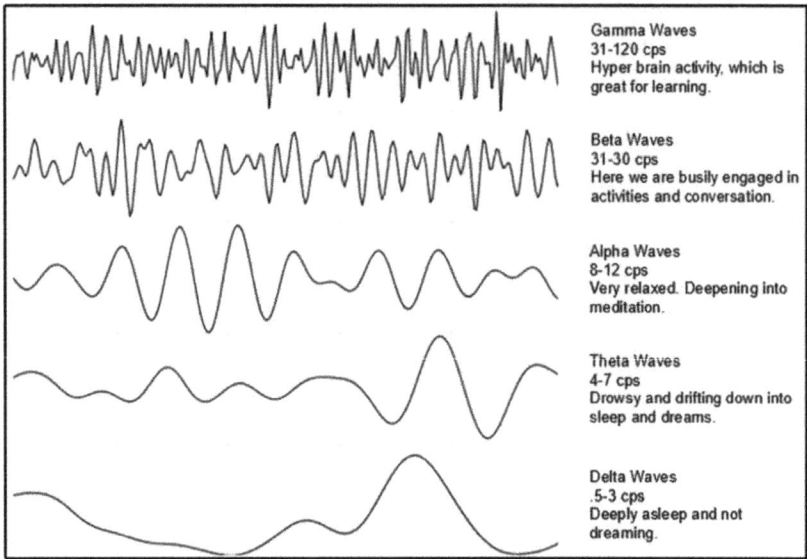

Figure 10.1: Relative frequencies of brain waves
Source:[154]

Gamma Waves

Gamma waves are probably the least understood frequency. They are also the most recently discovered frequency and are difficult to detect. It is considered that they are involved in both higher processing tasks and cognitive functioning. The more intelligent you are, the stronger the gamma waves.

The waves operate in a frequency range from 40 to 100 cycles per second. Unusually, at a 'gamma brainwave state' neurons fire together at the same time.

---

[154] http://mbyl.hubpages.com/hub/What-are-Gamma-Brain-Waves-How-to-produce-more-Gamma-Waves-with-Meditation#slide8522567

Counter-intuitively meditation, notably Mindfulness meditation, increases Gamma brain waves. This is counter-intuitive because the outcome of most forms of meditation is the lowering of brain frequencies into the Alpha / Theta range. Conversely, Gamma waves are associated with self-awareness and by increasing awareness through Mindfulness we also increase Gamma. This becomes a virtuous circle of cause and effect.

The belief is that gamma brain waves play a role in creating the unity of conscious perception which increases cognition. Research into this is still ongoing, but it is suggested gamma waves allow us to survive in a complex world; for instance, by being aware of the traffic and pedestrians around us as we commute to work. When a stimulus introduces potential danger, for example an oncoming bus, we instantly bring it into conscious control in order to respond.

The somewhat tricky question is: How do two brain waves of different frequencies co-exist with each other at the same time?

There is a parallel synergy between the Gamma and other frequencies upon sensory–cognitive input. This leads to the coexistence and cooperative action of these interwoven and interacting sub-mechanisms, so shaping the integrative brain functions.[155] This is because the brain does not exist in a single state of being as it would have been if two rhythms did not co-exist. Its dynamic and complex nature necessitate the intermingling of different aspects of the brain oscillations.

In simpler terms, the 40 Hz plus gamma wave is important for the binding of our senses in relation to our perception. For instance, when you are looking at something different parts of the brain register its

---

[155] Bașar, E. and Guntekin, B. (2013) Review of Delta, Theta, alpha, beta and gamma response oscillations in neuropsychiatric disorders. Suppl. Clin. Neurophysiol., Vol. 62, Ch. 2,

size, colour, and other features and Gamma unifies the information. Unsurprisingly then, it has been found that individuals who are mentally challenged and have learning disabilities tend to have lower gamma activity than average.

Beta Waves

This is the most rapid wave pattern, the pattern of normal waking consciousness. Beta is associated with concentration, arousal, alertness, and cognition. 'At its highest, most rapid levels, though, Beta is associated with anxiety, disharmony, and disease. Perhaps the ability to slow yourself down from those levels might be beneficial.'[156]

Operating at 14 to 30/35 cycles per second, this is our waking rhythm and will arise out of a focus on the world and life around us, but if we are emotionally agitated, this will increase to 40 cycles per second. High Beta waves, over 21 cycles per second, without Alpha waves are associated with stress, anxiety, high blood pressure, and similar issues.

Consistently high Beta levels reduce our immune system's effectiveness, enabling physical debilitation or illness to occur. At very high Beta levels (approaching 30 cycles per second) we become fidgety, restless and unfocussed on any one thing for long. Our mind will be pushing for an avenue to release this pent-up adrenalin.

'In most people, the right or left hemisphere of their brain is usually more dominant, a phenomenon called brain

------

[156] Centerpointe Research Institute Retrieved 24 March 2008 from http://www.centerpointe.com/

lateralization. As the amount of Beta brain wave levels increases, the brainwaves from both sides of the brain become increasingly out-of-phase.

In contrast, when your brainwaves slow down, both sides of your brain start to synchronize and communicate more with each other. Your neurons and brain cells start to fire synchronously in a coordinated manner.[157]

Given that Beta sharpens our responses and keeps us alert, we may think Beta is the most vital state in our survival toolkit. Beta-driven responses are immediate to what we interpret (usually wrongly) as life and death situations. Decisions made in Beta can be reactive and defensive, rather than collaborative and constructive.

Of course, Beta is important, but it can also keep us edgy and stressed out! Without realising it, we can easily spend most of our time in Beta and suffer many negative psychological and physical side effects as a result. So, the long-term effects of operating in Beta can be destructive.

Alpha Waves

'As you become more relaxed, your brain wave activity slows into what is called an Alpha brain wave pattern. Alpha patterns vary from deep Alpha, a state of deep relaxation often referred to as the twilight state between sleep and waking, to the higher end of Alpha which is a more focused yet still very relaxed state. When you are absorbed in a good book (or a television show) you are probably in Alpha. Alpha is often associated with what is known

---

[157] Guide to self Help Techniques Retrieved 24 March 2008 from http://www.guide-to-self-help-techniques.com/Beta-brainwaves.html

as 'super learning' —the ability to learn, process, store and recall large amounts of information quickly and efficiently.[158]

We can create Alpha waves by closing our eyes and un-focussing our mind. Our brain waves will pulse at a frequency of 8 to 13 cycles per second. Alpha waves are associated with feelings of relaxation and calmness. Alpha is sometimes described as the daydream state as most daydream activity occurs in us while in Alpha.

'Alpha rhythms are reported to be derived from the white matter of the brain. The white matter can be considered the part of the brain that connects all parts with each other. Alpha is a common state for the brain and occurs whenever a person is alert (it is a marker for alertness and sleep), but not actively processing information. They are strongest over the occipital (back of the head) cortex and also over [the] frontal cortex. Alpha has been linked to extroversion (introverts show less), creativity (creative subjects show Alpha when listening and coming to a solution for creative problems), and mental work. When our Alpha is within normal ranges, we tend to also experience good moods, see the world truthfully, and have a sense of calmness. Alpha is one of the brain's most important frequencies to learn and use information taught in the classroom and on the job.

You can increase Alpha by closing your eyes or deep breathing or decrease Alpha by thinking or calculating. Alpha-Theta training can create an increase in sensation, abstract thinking and self-control.[159]

[158] Centerpointe Research Institute Retrieved 24 March 2008 from http://www.centerpointe.com/
[159] Crossroads Institute retrieved 1 September 2007 from http://www.crossroadsinstitute.org/eeg.html

Alpha is the bridge that links the conscious and subconscious mind. You may also recall that when in a previous chapter we looked at the characteristics that so-called lucky people were exhibiting, they seem to reflect some of those found in an Alpha state of mind. Our mind switches into Alpha level during the day so that we're able to draw the memories stored in our subconscious mind into our conscious, thinking mind (Beta) where they can be remembered, processed, interpreted, and used.

Interesting Fact [160]

> Have you ever noticed that most people's eyes always look up every time they're trying to remember something?
>
> Researchers have discovered that every time your eyes look up about 30°, the brain momentarily generates Alpha brain wave patterns.
>
> If you close your eyes and look up behind your eyelids, the Alpha brain waves are even stronger. It's been proven that closing your eyes increases Alpha brainwaves.
>
> Western scientists still don't fully understand why this happens; however, spiritual teachers and Eastern philosophers explain that this is because you're accessing your subconscious through one of your chakras (situated roughly between your eyes).

Alpha waves are the healing frequency – when you are ill this is where your mind finds its best state and you become, to varying degrees, slower and more lethargic.

---

[160] Guide to self-help techniques Retrieved 1 September 2007 from http://www.guide-to-self-help-techniques.com/brain-wave.html

In Alpha we naturally have a better command of life, our health, and our moods. The Alpha dimension has a complete set of sensing faculties; in Alpha we can think more clearly, consider responses and perhaps make more creative decisions, with better long-term results. [161]

Alpha is our peaceful haven. It is a state we can visit, while fully conscious, that will always give us relief from stress. It overcomes insomnia and generates creativity, emotional flexibility and our capacity to remain calm and open in the face of tough decisions.

In Alpha we are at our most productive because we are fully awake, yet completely relaxed.

Sub-band low Alpha:[162] Pulsing with a frequency of 8 to 10 cycles per second leads to an inner awareness of self, mind/body integration, balance.

Sub-band high Alpha: Pulsing with a frequency of 10 to 12 cycles per second leads to centring, healing, and mind/body connection.

Another interesting benefit of Alpha and Theta brain waves is that they help improve our intuition and psychic abilities – or perhaps place us in a climate where we will experience synchronicity as we become consciously aware of the universe. Have you ever thought of a friend and then receive a phone call from them the next instant, or accidentally bump into them the next time you go out? This is because Alpha is the link between the conscious and subconscious mind, while Theta (below) is the realm of the subconscious and intuition. So, if our Alpha and Theta brain wave patterns are strong enough, it's a lot

[161] Silence of Music, retrieved 1 September 2007 fromhttp://www.silenceofmusic. com/articles/brainwaves1.html

[162] Crossroads Institute retrieved 1 September 2007 from http://www.crossroad-sinstitute.org/eeg.html

easier for intuitive messages from our subconscious or inner mind to reach our conscious mind. [163]

We need to balance Beta with Alpha to create optimum outcomes for wellbeing, inspiration, and effect.

Theta Waves

'Slower still are Theta waves. Theta is best known as the brain wave state of dreaming sleep, but it is also associated with a number of other beneficial states, including increased creativity, some kinds of super learning, increased memory abilities, and what are called integrative experiences (in which we make broadly-based positive changes in the way we see ourselves, others, or a certain life situation). 'Ah-ha!' experiences, where you suddenly 'get it,' have an insight, or a great idea suddenly comes to you, are accompanied by bursts of Theta waves in your brain. Critical and often self-sabotaging filters of the left brain are bypassed in a Theta state, and that [means that] in terms of making positive changes in beliefs or habit patterns, a lot of work gets done very quickly.' And best of all, Theta is also a state of tremendous stress relief. In the slower Theta brain wave pattern, the brain makes lots of relaxing endorphins that really do...melt your stress away.'[164]

Theta has a frequency of approximately 4 to 7 cycles per second and you can induce Theta with meditation; however, as you will no doubt have discovered, this can lead to drowsiness or even sleep. Lucid dreams are more prone to occur in Theta. The mind is in a twilight state and

---

[163] Guide to self-help techniques.com Retrieved 24 March 2008 from http://www. guide-to-self-help-techniques.com/brain-wave.html

[164] Centerpointe Research Institute Retrieved 24 March 2008 from http://www. centerpointe.com/

is prone to free association resulting in amazing mental images.[165] It reflects the state between wakefulness and sleep. Theta relates to the subconscious mind.

Delta Waves

'The slowest brain wave pattern is Delta, the brain wave pattern of dreamless sleep. Generally, people are asleep in Delta, but there is evidence that it is possible to remain alert in this state —a very deep, trance-like, non-physical state you'll have to experience to appreciate. 'In certain Delta frequencies the brain releases many highly beneficial substances, including human growth hormone, which we ordinarily make in decreasing quantities as we get older, resulting in many aging symptoms including loss of muscle tone, increased weight gain, loss of stamina, and many diseases associated with aging.'

Delta has a frequency of about 0.5 to 4 cycles per second. Delta is our experience when in a deep sleep. People do not dream when they are in Delta sleep. We *increase* Delta waves in order to decrease our awareness of the physical world. We also access information in our unconscious mind through Delta when, with training, we go into a trance or deeply relaxed state.

---

[165] Scientific Audio Resources Retrieved 1 September 2007 from http://www.rainfall.com/cdroms/default.htm

Figure 10.2: Four categories of brain wave patterns[166]

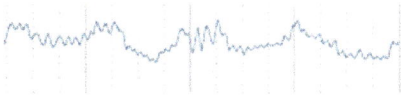

Beta (14-30 Hz)

Concentration, arousal, alertness, cognition

Higher levels associated with anxiety, unease, feelings of separation, fight or flight

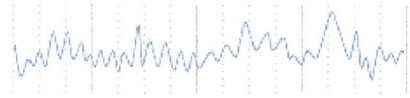

Alpha (8-13.9 Hz)

Relaxation, super learning, relaxed focus, light trance, increased serotonin production

Pre-sleep, pre-waking drowsiness, meditation, beginning of access to unconscious mind

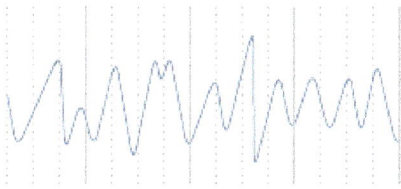

Theta (4-7.9 Hz)

Dreaming sleep (REM sleep)
Increased production of catecholamines (vital for learning and memory), increased creativity

Integrative, emotional experiences, potential change in behaviour, increased retention of learned material

Hypnagogic imagery, trance, deep meditation, access to unconscious mind

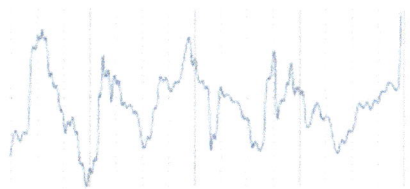

Delta (.1-3.9 Hz)

Dreamless sleep
Human growth hormone released

Deep, trance-like, non-physical state, loss of body awareness

Access to unconscious and 'collective unconscious' mind, greatest 'push' to brain when induced with Holosync®

---

[166] Centerpointe Research Institute Retrieved 24 March 2008 from http://www. centerpointe.com/

It is said that, with training, the brain can operate in more than one state at the same time, in different parts of the brain.

Change your brain change your life expectancy.

Traditionally, Western biomedicine has shunned the study of personal experiences and emotions in relation to physical health. In recent years, however, there has been a sharp shift in mainstream academia and in health systems around the world. The state of a person's mind has become the focus of research with a view to slowing ageing, lengthening life and reducing anxiety and pain. One of the reasons for this has been the work of Australian Nobel prize winner, Dr. Elizabeth Blackburn, who:

> '.... *discovered a repeating DNA motif that acts as a protective cap (to Chromosome tips). The caps, dubbed telomeres, were subsequently found on human chromosomes too. They shield the ends of our chromosomes each time our cells divide and the DNA is copied, but they wear down with each division. In the 1980s, working with graduate student Carol Greider at the University of California, Berkeley, Blackburn discovered an enzyme called telomerase that can protect and rebuild telomeres. Even so, our telomeres dwindle over time. And when they get too short, our cells start to malfunction and lose their ability to divide – a phenomenon that is now recognised as a key process in ageing.*[167]

Stress reduces the length of telomeres and subsequent studies have shown that elderly men whose telomeres shortened over two-and-a-half years were three times as likely to die from cardiovascular disease

---

[167] Jo Marchant, *Can meditation really slow ageing?*

in the subsequent nine years as those whose telomeres stayed the same length or got longer.

In more recent times Dr Blackburn has been involved in trials that have suggested that one of the most effective interventions, apparently capable of slowing the erosion of telomeres – and even lengthening them again – is meditation.[168]

Meditation, twenty-five years ago, was seen by any serious medical researcher as a step too far into the bizarre; however, in the twenty-first century 'researchers have developed secularised – or non-religious – practices such as Mindfulness-based stress reduction and Mindfulness-based cognitive therapy and reported a range of health effects from lowering blood pressure and boosting immune responses to warding off depression; and the past few years have seen a spurt of neuroscience studies, like Lazar's, showing that even short courses of meditation can forge structural changes in the brain.'[169] Such meditation changes our thought processes as well.

A final word

What has been outlined above strongly supports The IDEA that we can change our state of being through our thought processes, even as our thought processes change the experiences of our lives. This is because the incredible physical structure of our brain is like a piece of malleable marble waiting to be sculpted. We are the Leonardo da Vinci of the sculpture that is carved, because *'the brain is now known to be physically shaped by contributions from both our genes and our experience,*

---

[168] Ibid
[169] Ibid

working together.[170] It is plastic, malleable and we can shape it. We can do this because we can control the levels and types of stimulation to our brain and, therefore, the type of synaptic connections we create.

---

[170] The Surgeon General retrieved 21 July 2008 from http://www.surgeongeneral. gov/library/mentalhealth/chapter2/sec1.html

CHAPTER 11

The Pygmalion Effect - Expectation Theory – or 'when people try and tell you who you are, don't believe them'

What is the Pygmalion Effect?

I am not who I think I am, I am not who you think I am, I am who I think you think I am (Robert Schuller).

MEETING THE EXPECTATIONS THAT OUR parents, our teachers, our leaders, set for us is something that we learned to do in our early childhood years. These expectations drive our decisions and affect the directions we take in life. One problem we face in choosing our own path and opening up our paradigms is that much of who we are and what we believe about ourselves has been shaped by the expectations of others. The opening quote may sound convoluted, but when you think on it you see that it is so true.

As psychologist Robert Rosenthal puts it, *'what one person expects of another can come to serve as a self-fulfilling prophecy.'*

> **Unconsciously we tend to live life to a greater or lesser degree as chameleons.**

Unconsciously, we live life to a greater or lesser degree as chameleons. We change our nature, and our responses, to match what we believe are the expectations of others. Have you ever been away from your parents, or a particular group of friends, for some long while and then, when you see them again, you slip back into old ways of behaving around them?

Our belief in the possibility of change, together with our acceptance of the possibilities afforded by the inner workings of the brain and the external laws of the universe, can only be realised if we have the strength to stand against these conforming pressures and expectations. Most of the time, we are totally unaware of our conforming nature. This is because the synaptic connections in our brains that lead us to conform have long been established.

When we were children, we sort of knew what we were good at, even if others didn't. The tragedy of growing older is that, for many people, that clarity faded with the passage of those early years - childhood, teen years and then adult life - as we started listening to the world around us more closely than we did to our authentic inner being. We lost confidence in who we felt we really were and what we could do.

This loss of confidence in ourselves can mean that as we grow into the autumn of life (psychologically much earlier for some than for others) and find ourselves in a rapidly changing world with shifting values, we try to micromanage our external environment to avoid the challenge of change. We would sooner do this than change our thinking, our attitudes, and our behaviour to better match those changes occurring around us.

This is because it can be distressing when we now find that the changes we see around us do not match our beliefs. Those beliefs were largely formed up by the prevailing wisdom of those around us in our younger life and by the culture we were immersed in, and that resultant *wisdom* has been the bedrock of our existence. As an example, it took over a generation to change attitudes to women, to gay rights, to the environment and, for not a few people, some of these and other issues can remain irreconcilable with their value/cultural base embedded by societal pressures of earlier years.

As a result, rather than confronting the inconsistencies within our acquired beliefs, it is more convenient to shape our external surroundings to align with our internal perspectives. We achieve this by:

- being highly selective in choosing the individuals we associate with;
- making deliberate choices about the places we visit; and
- controlling our activities, as well as our reading and viewing materials.

By doing so, we attempt to avoid inner conflicts that arise when we encounter new information contradicting our existing beliefs, ideas, or values. Instead, we hold on to our internal mental frameworks that define our identity, values, and perception of the world. We find solace in their familiarity. We may express our views fervently, particularly among like-minded groups, as we strive to impose our worldview on others and thus, the cycle continues across generations.

It all begins in our early years, when we were very vulnerable to the perceptions of those adults around us. Their values, beliefs, and insights, whether spoken or unspoken, shaped our neural pathways, creating responsive behaviour. Other people's perception of us also can, and does, shape our performance. As a young child, I must have been about six. I was repeatedly told by my father, who was watching me play with a Meccano set, that I was mechanically incapable. The consequence was that I avoided anything mechanical, and it was many years before I discovered I was actually as capable as the next person.

Let me ask you – did your parents, teammates, or teachers ever tell you that you would never be able to do something, or imply that you would never amount to anything? Did these thoughts in some way find confirmation from friends, workmates, bosses, or others as you travelled through your life? Often such confirmations are subliminal; they are not stated, and they exist below the threshold of your consciousness. It should be noted that positive affirmation by significant adults works with equal force.

Let me give you an example of how this plays out in real life:

In the 1960s, two researchers lied to prove students would rise to meet their teachers' expectations. They undertook a series of experiments on school children to demonstrate that reality was changed by the expectations of others. The two researchers were psychologist, Robert Rosenthal, and school principal, Lenore Jacobson. In particular, their study showed that if teachers were led to expect enhanced performance from some children by being told, for instance, that their children were A-stream students, then the children did indeed show that enhancement. In some cases, such an improvement was about twice that shown by other children in the same class. The teachers in the experiments were not aware that their expectations had been artificially raised or lowered by third parties. What was discovered was that consequential unconscious influences can be both detrimental, as well as beneficial, depending on which label the teacher has been given for the child.[171]

This is known as the Pygmalion Effect.

> **'The difference between a flower girl and a lady is not in the way she acts, but in the way she is treated.'**

Rosenthal and Jacobson borrowed the term Pygmalion Effect from the play Pygmalion by George Bernard Shaw in which a professor's high expectations radically transformed the educational performance of a 'lower-class girl'.[172] In the musical version, My Fair Lady, Eliza Doolittle sums this up by saying: *The difference between a flower girl and a lady is not in the way she acts, but in the way she is treated.'*

The effect is sometimes seen as a form of self-fulfilling prophecy lived out at many levels of our everyday lives and in our societies. It is also experienced when we encounter people who are trying to reshape who they are and those around them persist in relating to them as who they once were.

This can result in their failure to achieve the change they seek.

This is most obvious when individuals are trying to give up addictive habits, change their diets, reduce their drinking, or break free from a criminal past. It is also encountered when individuals have undergone counselling and who then try to relinquish past patterns of behaviour, such as being a victim or feeling needy.

[171] Wikipedia recovered 3 November 2007 from http://en.wikipedia.org/wiki/Pygmalion_effect#Rosenthal-Jacobson_study

[172] History of education, Retrieved 3 November 2007 from http://fcis.oise.utoronto.ca/~daniel_sc/assignment1/1968rosenjacob.html

The Pygmalion in the classroom study was followed by many other school-based studies that examined these mechanisms in detail from different perspectives. Prominent among the works conducted by American scholars on this subject are *'Student social class and teacher expectations: The self-fulfilling prophecy in ghetto education'* (Ray Rist 1970), *'Social class and the hidden curriculum of work'* (Jean Anyon 1980), *'Keeping track: How schools structure inequality'* (Jeannie Oakes 1984), and *'Failing at fairness: How America's schools cheat girls,'* (Myra Sadker and David Sadker 1995).[173]

By way of another example, Christiane Northup, M.D., writes in her book *Women's Bodies, Women's Wisdom* of the Tarahumara Indians of Mexico. This is a group known for their running ability. Routinely, certain members of the tribe ran the equivalent of a marathon or more every day; however, the most intriguing aspect of their culture was that they believed the best runners were those in their 60s. She tells of how Dr Deepak Chopra (an endocrinologist and internationally-recognised authority on how consciousness works), reporting on an experiment by a team of researchers, showed that the best lung capacity, cardiovascular fitness and endurance were indeed found in runners in their sixties. What Dr Chopra pointed out is that for this belief to translate into physical reality, the entire tribe had to believe it.[174]

What does this mean for us?

Well, mostly, the world around us tends only to be concerned about what or who we are relative to their requirements. Faced with the world's indifference, we have two options, either to:

---

[173] History of education, Retrieved 3 November 2007 from http://fcis.oise.uto-ronto.ca/~daniel_sc/assignment1/1968rosenjacob.html

[174] Northrup, C. 1998 *Women's Bodies Women's Wisdom* Judy Piatkus Publishers Ltd London p489

- resign ourselves to a life designed by the needs and expectations of those around us, whether spouse, parent, employer, friend, or work colleague; or
- learn to recognise, and subsequently harness, our unique strengths, aligning them with our individual life purpose. In the process, we enhance our authenticity.[175]

An American school in New Jersey has featured on a number of American national shows because of its unique approach. This school is the Purnell School for Girls. It had as its focus those girls for whom the Pygmalion Effect had worked to the detriment of their previous lives and well-being. Unashamedly, Purnell accepted: *'girls who will be happier and more successful in a smaller setting where their talents and personalities are celebrated and they are not lost in the crowd. A Purnell girl may have a strong interest in the arts, may feel she marches to the beat of a different drum, or may want to get off the bench and onto the playing fields. It is also a school for girls who are still trying to discover their potential, or who may have found success elusive in the past. A Purnell girl is someone who cares about her future and wants to make the most of her high school years. Sometimes a Purnell girl may have felt lost, misunderstood or unnoticed in a former setting.'*

Sadly, the school officially closed following the 2020–21 academic school year citing *'challenges related to the competitive landscape.'*

I should add that I have no connection to this school, but isn't that a powerful vision statement which changed the experience of life for those girls fortunate enough to have attended that academy?

---

[175] Personal authenticity is often defined as being true and honest with oneself and others, having a credibility in one's words and behavior

Another example which touched me is occurring in Uganda, Central Africa.

Uganda has endured brutal dictators, the scourge of civil war, and the deadly AIDS epidemic. An estimated two million children in Uganda have been orphaned by these calamities, 880,000 of them as a result of AIDS alone (UNAIDS stats). In 1994, a couple by the name of Gary and Marilyn Skinner started an unusual program in Kampala, Uganda, the heartland of Africa. Horrified at the devastation of AIDS, wars, and child soldiers in Africa, and the consequent millions of orphaned children whose lives were shattered, who felt worthless and abandoned by God and man, and who became vulnerable to the world around them, the Skinners developed a work that is unusual in its paradigm. This work is called Watoto. What makes this work unusual is that it seeks not only to house, clothe, feed, and educate these children, but to change the way they see themselves. Not as recipients of a handout, of another worthwhile Western-based intervention strategy, but as being equipped to be future leaders in their devastated country. The fundraising slogan of the initiative is *'Rescue a Child, Raise a Leader, Rebuild a Nation.'* Their written expectation is expressed as follows:

'Look at a Watoto child and see a leader, equipped to make a lasting impact in their community and on Uganda.'

When we are not aligned with our natural design and human potential we have an internal dissonance between our inner core beliefs about ourselves and our external conforming practices and behaviour.

The ability to reprint our brain to overcome the handicap of our early lives, as well as other people's expectations, is not confined to our childhood years. It is never too late to recognise what has taken place and how our attitudes towards ourselves, and others, have been shaped (warped?) by another's beliefs and expectations and so begin to make internal changes that allow us to open the door to what life truly can offer us.

We are not a body that has a soul – we are a soul that has a body!

To balance the Pygmalion Effect – be authentic

'One of the greatest moments in anybody's developing experience is when he no longer tries to hide from himself but determines to get acquainted with himself as he really is.'[176] Norman Vincent Peale

If the Pygmalion Effect is rising or falling in line with other people's expectations, then being authentic is possibly an opposite, as it calls on each of us to be true to who we really are in our thoughts, feelings and actions. It involves aligning our behaviour and choices with our values, beliefs and identity, rather than trying to conform to societal expectations or pretending to be someone else.

It can be difficult to deliberately change our expectations of others, but we can consciously change our behaviour.

> **The person, who holds the greatest influence over your behaviour, is yourself.**
> Dr. Jean Caldow

Each one of us has a special and unique purpose in life; a purpose supported by the resources of the universe.

The key to our success in realising that purpose is developing a true alignment with our natural design, failing which the brain will substitute an alternative alignment. That

---

[176] https://www.brainyquote.com/quotes/norman_vincent_peale_159739

alternative alignment may be that of the culture in which we are immersed. This is unsurprising since it is our culture, along with our family, that shaped our values, gave us our learning, our sense of morality, our ideas, and our manners and so, on from birth.

Yet, every culture is different and different cultural activities produce different outcomes in people's lives. This very difference suggests that no culture is complete in and of itself because one of the greatest problems many of us face, as reflected in the Pygmalion Effect, is that we believe our culture's implicit interpretation of our life, reality and purpose.

Our cultural values and mores have been conveyed to us by parents and reinforced by the media and those around us in all aspects of life. This self-reinforcing culture may be the culture of the nation we live in or a subgroup we belong to. Our view of ourselves and the world around us is unlikely to be truly aligned with our natural design and inherent potential.

When that happens, we have an internal dissonance between our inner core beliefs about ourselves and our external conforming practices and behaviour.

This dissonance arises because we are responding to our external environment and other people's voices and opinions, rather than to that intuitive voice in us which would guide us according to our inner values. In this state, we become 'chameleon like' as we seek to blend into others' expectations and the surrounding environment.

Consequently, we can find ourselves in relationships, at parties, or in workplaces where we have a vague sense of unease, an unease that we cannot quite place, all because we are not being authentic. There is a tension between who we are by design and what we find ourselves doing.

How can we identify some areas where we lack authenticity?

When we are not totally authentic, our principles are compromised and we tend to live compartmentalised lives with differing principles governing our behaviour. For instance, there is our home life, our work life, our private self, our public self, and so on. For instance:

- When you are at work does your work self shout and get angry the same way that perhaps you might do in your home life? Or vice versa?
- Is your behaviour in public the same as that in private?
- Do you privately think one thing and publicly say another?
- Do you get involved in behaviours that you would prefer not to? How many people go along with a bully in the workplace in making fun of a colleague in case they become the next target?
- Do you drink with boys or party with the girls when you really want to be at home with your partner?

Of course, for different reasons, this may be true occasionally. When, however, this is largely the case we need to recognise that each behaviour, to a greater and lesser degree, is not authentically us. Don't accept the lowest common denominator of behaviour – change your behaviour and raise the bar to the highest standard, matching your principles.

Being authentic is essential if we are to successfully increase the level of our consciousness and awareness in our lives. Being authentic requires that we are honest with ourselves, as well as with those around us. Being authentic often involves facing and embracing our fears, insecurities, and shadows. This journey of self-discovery and self-acceptance leads to personal growth and transformation. As we become more conscious of our inner landscape, we can let go of limiting beliefs, patterns and behaviours that hinder our growth, allowing us to unlock our full potential.

Authenticity is crucial for increasing consciousness and awareness in our lives. It supports self-awareness, alignment with our values, the removal of masks and illusions, deeper connections with others, and inner transformation. By living authentically, we create the space for greater self-realisation and expanded consciousness.

The strain of acting out of an illusionary self all the time can crush our spirits and steal our joy. A lack of authenticity will often undermine other's trust in you and so the integrity and strength of your relationships; it will also limit your leadership and diminish opportunity.

> **"The privilege of a lifetime is to become who you truly are."**
> C.G. Jung

Sue Fitzmaurice provides the following guidelines to achieving authenticity:

- be more concerned with truth than opinions;
- be sincere and do not pretend;
- be free from hypocrisy - walk your talk;
- know who you are and be that person;
- do not fear others seeing your vulnerabilities;
- be confident to walk away from situations where you can't be yourself;
- be awake to your own feelings;
- be free from others' opinions of you; and
- accept and love yourself.[177]

---

[177] http://www.goodreads.com/quotes/tag/authenticity

In considering success and the Law of Attraction, know that *'you can only give wholehearted commitment when all your objectives are aligned, and your principles are not compromised.'*[178] and that wholehearted ongoing commitment is needed for a successful authentic life.

Therefore, the starting point to being an authentic person is to be honest with ourselves. Until we are honest with ourselves, we cannot trust aspects of ourselves in different situations. With honesty comes insight – there is no hiding and so your self-awareness increases.

One reality of personal dishonesty is that we destine ourselves to repeat experiences in our lives. This is because as the truth in those experiences is suppressed, it will resurface in different contexts until we recognise, acknowledge and deal with it.

One of my favourite films is a film called *Groundhog Day* with Bill Murray and Andie MacDowell. It recounts the story of a TV meteorologist, Phil Connors, his producer Rita, and cameraman Larry, from the fictional Pittsburgh television station WPBH-TV9, who travel to Punxsutawney, Pennsylvania, to cover the annual festivities (which in real life, as in the movie, holds a major celebration for Groundhog Day).

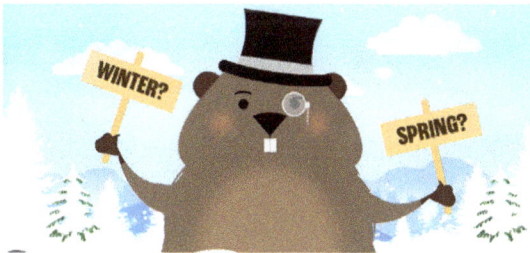

179

---

[178] Crofts, N. 2003, *Authentic: How to make a living by being yourself* Capstone Publishing Ltd UK.

[179] News10 ABC

The story recounts Phil Connors reliving one day over and over, until he finally becomes an authentic man by working through the drivers of his behaviour. He became aligned as a personality and freed from the trailing tendrils of past experiences that biased his behaviour and life. In so doing he enhanced his own human understanding which, in turn, made him an appreciated and beloved man in the town.

We may have our own version of Groundhog Day which sees us repeating patterns of behaviour, but unless we are aware of those patterns in our life nothing changes. We can, however, use therapy, meditation or some other strategy that will lead us to a greater awareness of who we really are – our authentic selves, and so change.

Until such time as we do become self-aware, much of the content of The IDEA can only apply in a limited fashion.

CHAPTER 12

The Ecology of Being

'I am because we are.' [180]

'A person is a person through other persons.' [181]

T HE PHILOSOPHICAL DARKNESS OF THIS scientific age is finally
shifting. For over one hundred years, the predominant Western
philosophical approach saw us as individual rational entities, with
autonomous wills and intellects, forging our separate destinies in an
atomised, mechanistic world. We have become increasingly separated
in all dimensions of existence from the community of being that
pervades the earth and the universe around us.

So much so that some have argued that God is dead and there is no
logical answer to the dilemmas of life that we face, for all is chaotic,
irrational, and absurd.

---

[180] African aphorism (Lewin & Regine 2000 xi)
[181] African proverb

Jacques Monod, writing on this perspective, had this to say:

'If he accepts this message in its full significance, man must at last wake out of his millenary dream and discover his total solitude, his fundamental isolation. He must realise that, like a gypsy, he lives on the boundary of an alien world; a world that is deaf to his music, and as indifferent to his hopes as it is to his suffering or his crimes.' [182]

Unsurprisingly then, many of us live in private alienation even as we are exposed to the broader world, in all its extremities, through the media. In fact, the stupendous amount of information fed to us on an historically unprecedented scale has led to our world seeming less certain and less ordered. This has led to a personal sense of disempowerment, causing a psychological withdrawal and a spiritual crisis - the *God is dead* syndrome. Authenticity in this atomised existence is reflected in a need to embrace its futility and this has resulted in the smothering of the awareness of our mortality with materialistic narcissism as we create malls for our consumerist souls.

> **Our humanity is fundamentally rooted in our social connections .... our individual growth and fulfillment are intimately tied to the well-being of the community around us.**

In more recent times though, with concepts such as that of the collective unconscious, the Gaia hypothesis, the interpenetration of eastern teachings, the postulation of Chaos Theory, the development of Quantum Physics, and the establishment of systems thinking and dissipative structures (the list could go on), there are too many contradictions for that paradigm of nihilism

---

[182] Monod, J. 1970 *The ethics of knowledge and the socialist ideal*, Chance and Necessity publ. Collins, 1970

to be sustainable in the twenty-first century, let alone to remain unchallenged.

Increasingly, there is an awareness that we are inter-dependent. Instead of holding to a theory of being (ontology) that is individualistic, we can now see one that talks of our interdependence within a participatory universe. We are joint architects of our individual and collective futures. At its most fundamental level, we can recognise the overlapping and interweaving of symbiotic relationships and similarities at all levels of existence. At its most publicised point, we see in the looming issue of climate change an example of the reality of such interlinked systems.

Where such relationships were always evident in nature to those who were interested, these connections are now widely acknowledged as being the case at all levels of creation, including the intangibles of psychology, physics, and the unseen worlds. The connections form, if you like, the synapses of the universe and, like synapses of the brain, there are gaps between the parts which are bridged by electro/chemical packages.

Universally we appreciate the power and the role of the unconscious in its interface with these unseen realms of life, as The IDEA outlines. We are not only *not alone,* but we have been given the tools to make meaning and purpose out of the complexity of our existence through the web of life which is our medium of relationship with creation.

The engine of life is linkage

Much of this book, so far, has focussed on us as individuals, but in truth we live in the context of other human beings and, indeed, of the whole of the surrounding creation. The engine of life is linkage, nothing is inseparable.

> **We live in a world of probabilities, not a probability of things, but a probability of interconnections.**

In the chapter on Quantum Physics, we saw that the world could not be understood by the traditional Newtonian physics, which tried to reduce all physical phenomena to its individual properties of matter. In Newton's terms, the world was a perfect machine. Newton's theories were the arbiters of scientific thinking for centuries; then in the 1920s a radical new theory came on the scene – Quantum Theory.

Quantum Theory changed our thinking as it forced us to recognise that we live in a world of probabilities, not a probability of things, but a probability of interconnections. It demonstrated that there are no isolated building blocks; rather, there exists a complex web of relationships.[183] Quantum Theory points to the profound interconnectedness at the heart of life.

We are familiar in these days of climate change with the word *ecology*. What you may not be aware of is that its origin is *oikos*, meaning *household*. And it is therefore a study of those things that interlink all the members of earth's household, human and non-human.

Our understanding of the inter-relationship between all living things and their environment is growing with each passing year. At the most obvious level, we recognise carnivores eat herbivores that eat plants which, because of photosynthesis, gives the herbivores energy. Plants depend on the minerals in the ground, the carbon dioxide in the air and the nitrogen fixing bacteria on their root systems, and so maintain and regulate the biosphere in which we live. This provides us with a virtuous circle of life; that is a circle of activities that reinforce life with positive results.

---

[183] Capra, F 1996 *The web of life* HarperCollins Publishers London p 30

So, there is a fundamental unity to life that links all levels of nature, from networks of cells to the food webs of ecosystems. Life is fundamentally 'one'. As the artist Henri Matisse put it:

When we speak of Nature, it is wrong to forget that we are ourselves a part of Nature. We ought to view ourselves with the same curiosity and openness with which we study a tree, the sky or a thought, because we too are linked to the entire universe.

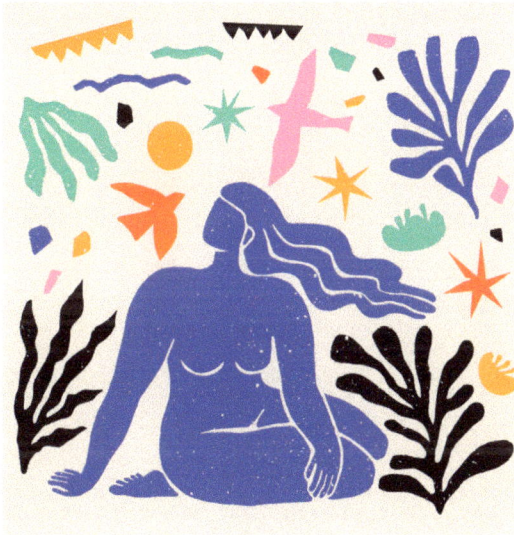

184

Such ecological expressions represent a profound shift in thinking from that of the past few centuries; a shift that has taken place in recent years yet is philosophically our starting point. We no longer see ourselves existing as singular individuals, separate from the world; we recognise we are part of a creational system, an interconnected web of life. Whereas before, we might not have been bothered by the activities of others, such as whether farmers sprayed plants and insects with DDT (think Rachel Carson and *The Silent Spring*), the

184 Freepic: Henry Matisse

reckless damming of waterways, fishing with dynamite, and so on; now we recognise that all of humanity's activities have a cascading impact that ultimately impinges on our world, our environment, our lives, and the lives of our children.

What we have described is the visible and, now that it has been pointed out to us, the self-evident truth about the natural ecology of the creation, but it goes further than this. There is in fact, no such thing as a singular idea or desire in life because everything is joined to everything else; while we may want to be singular, life is so interconnected that whatever we do, say, or even think, provides multiple responses in a connected environment. Nothing moves in a singular fashion.

A seventeenth century writer, John Donne, wrote a poem, *For Whom The Bell Tolls,* at a time when church bells were tolled for funerals. This poem illustrates his understanding of our interconnectedness. The following is an extract:

> *No man is an island, entire of itself; every man is a piece of the continent, a part of the main. If a clod be washed away by the sea, Europe is the less, as well as if a promontory were, as well as if a manor of thy friend's or of thine own were: any man's death diminishes me, because I am involved in mankind, and therefore never send to know for whom the bell tolls; it tolls for thee.*

Just as there is an external ecology of life in the world we inhabit, so there is also an inner ecology. This ecology of the mind links us to that outer world. How we perceive the outer world is selective, leading to a real time *interpretation* of what that outer world looks like. Earlier we discussed that as a species we think in patterns. We select information from the random bits that cross our sensory screen and create mental patterns filtered by our paradigms or prevailing beliefs, sometimes to good effect and sometimes to bad effect.

If, as the American physicist David Bohm suggests, the universe is characterised by a flow that integrates everything, then our individual thought forms are the equivalent of the still frames of an object in motion and we perceive reality through these static images.[185] Similarly, philosopher/scientist Gregory Bateson[186] suggests that the ecology of the mind is an ecology of pattern, information, and ideas that are embodied in things – in material forms.

So, our mind crosses our physical construct of the brain using the processes and patterns of thought. In this way our mind has an affinity for the world we live in, for that is the root of our sensory interpretation of life and its meaning. The resultant consciousness and awareness create connectivity between our inner and outer worlds.

If we can recognise that we are connected with everything else around us; that we are part of a larger system; that even in our thoughts we are part of a fabric of a web of life throughout this universe, then how much easier is it to also recognise that we will attract to us those things that vibrate with the same frequency as our individual thoughts, beliefs, and actions, as demonstrated in the next section.

Still, there is more... because we are a part of a larger fabric, then *collectively*, we can consciously create stronger outcomes for the big issues this world faces, the cure for cancer, for instance, or the way to peace. We can, in fact, *collectively* change our world; and that's something to be excited about!

Isn't there something a little scary in all this interconnectedness; a fear that we will lose our individual identity – causing us to cry from the

---

185 The Nature of Consciousness Retrieved 17 July 2008 from http://www.scaruffi.com/nature/consc3.html

186 Bateson, G. 1979, *Mind and Nature: A Necessary Unity* Bantam Books USA

heart, *what about me, as an individual?* There is indeed a tension between being one with the universe and maintaining our individual identity.

This may be resolved if we think about it this way:

- our identity is bound up in our personality; and
- our unity is reflected in our character and nature.

Regarding the second point, what I mean by this is that, over time, our character and nature are shaped as we become aware and responsive to the 'whole' that is around us. We are born helpless and are open to the environment, both human and non-human, around us. That environment will help shape and influence our character. This interconnection cuts two ways and can affect us both positively and negatively.

For instance, in times of recession, or even more so in times of depression, there is a general sense of difficulty and scarcity. Whether it's in relation to jobs, or more particularly money, there is a collective psychology which creates a collective energy. This is powerful as it is supported and loaded with that strong emotion, fear. This same collective psychology impels social moods, trends, and cultural expressions. This collective mood can impact the choices people make, the decisions they take, and the overall direction of societal trends.

> **Your thoughts are incredibly powerful - choose yours wisely.**
> Dr Joe Dispenza

Trends, whether they are fashion, music, or other cultural expressions, are influenced by collective psychology. People's desires for acceptance, identity, and connection drive them to seek common interests and align with popular trends, whether as groups, or communities or populations.

If thoughts become things, then consider how powerfully collective thoughts not only become things but can impact us. This concept underlies the Pygmalion Effect, as we have seen. All of us are affected. A sense of lack, or not enough, is coalescing (at the time of writing) as the global economy of the developed world appears to have hit some very troubled waters. We are a part of that collective energy, and we may be noticing even now our fear of 'not enough'. At other times, the collective energy pushes the good times to new heights and then bubbles form, whether in real estate prices or stock market prices. Individually, people borrow and spend as though there is no tomorrow because the collective belief is so ebulliently optimistic and then we are all affected when the bubble bursts and prices fall, usually spectacularly.

One writer illustrated the difficulty in our perceiving the existent networks surrounding us, by likening us to fish in the sea. For just as a fish is immersed in a sea of water – and is completely unaware of the substance that has always surrounded it – so are we immersed in a sea of unseen knowledge, connection and communication, one that we are only now beginning to comprehend and become aware of.[187]

Arthur Koestler, a twentieth century philosopher, refers to *'the universal hanging-together of things, their embeddedness in a universal matrix.'*[188] Many ecologists already subscribe to this deep sense of interrelation in the world. This is what the ancients called the *sympathy* of life.

And the concept of inter-relationship is not new.

---

[187] Jensen, A. and Westra, C. 2007 Twelve Ways to Consciously Create What You Want in 2007

[188] Physics and Consciousness Retrieved 8 February 2008 from http://www.star-stuffs.com/physcon2/shamanism.html

Dating back to around the third century BC Taoism, is a major school of thought arising out of China, has influenced its culture, art and religion. Taoist precepts form the foundations of such disparate disciplines as Acupuncture, Tai Chi, the I-Ch'ing, and Ju-Jitsu. A basic tenet of Taoist thought is that the operation of the human world should ideally be contiguous to, or touching, that of the natural order. This is because all facets of the world are interdependent, and we need to find harmony in the universe for whatever it is we are considering or undertaking.

In Tao lies the principle of Yin and Yang which adopt a polarity of approach to life – yet these two polar opposites are seen not as separate things, but as a part of a whole;[189] as complementary partners in a cosmic waltz. Yin, symbolised by the black swirl, represents darkness, femininity, stillness, and receptivity. Yang, the white swirl, embodies light, masculinity, activity, and assertion. It is symbolised by a circle divided into two halves by a curved line. The circle represents the interconnectedness of the world, particularly the natural world, and that the universe is governed by a cosmic duality, sets of two opposing and complementing principles or cosmic energies that can be observed in nature.

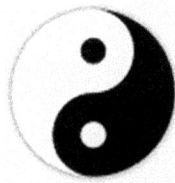

Now, picture these two forces swirling together, forming the iconic Taijitu symbol. It's a beautiful visual metaphor for their interdependence. Notice how each side holds a seed of the other – the black dot in the white, the white dot in the black. This symbolises their constant interplay, their dance of transformation.

---

[189] Watts, A. 1992 Tao: *The Watercourse Way* ARKANA Penguin Books NY USA

For most of us, the interconnection between ourselves and our family and friends and the workplace, exists as a given. Perhaps we need to do some work on recognising our interconnection with our local community, and ultimately to our entire planet. It is important to recognise that relationship, as an aspect of our being, is embedded in our nature.

Any thinking, or actions at any level of being, including spiritual, that alienates us from such recognition, will separate us from who we should be. Yet, as we have seen, there is a pull on our thinking in many directions, taking us away from being a part of a whole to being an individual whose shard of existence means life is precariously balanced on the vagaries of fortune.

It is almost universally agreed that there is a scientific basis for spirituality (without trying to define what that means any further). But the strictest evolutionary (almost Newtonian) theories that are put forward suggest that we are an accident of cause and effect in a mechanistic universe arising out of an algae-covered lake on a lonely planet, in a barren solar system, stuck in a lonely cosmos. This narrative creates in us a sense of separateness, aloneness, isolation and alienation. This view of separateness from each other and from the creation around us is highly destructive to our psyche, to our personal wellbeing and, indeed, to the wellbeing of those around us and the planet on which we live.

If the Newtonian perspective were the case, then the only question remaining, as the French author Albert Camus suggested is, 'Why not suicide right away and be done with it?'[190]

---

[190] The International Fiction Review Retrieved 18 May 2008 from http://www.lib. unb.ca/Texts/IFR/bin/get.cgi?directory=Vol.26/&filename=Stoltzfus.htm

As I have sought to briefly illustrate, every aspect of our world works on the basis that we are interconnected.

What does this matter or mean to us?

As within, so without

Some of us have become so addicted to the material world and to the amount of stuff we own, that we can find ourselves separated from the ecological whole. More than that, our *focus* on acquisition hinders us from personal development and our spiritual development, so that even at the simplest level we are not internally integrated. Just as we can damage the environment around us, we can pollute and damage the internal environment of our soul.

From the outset I have stated that:

Our beliefs define our reality.

It is a common misconception that this means all we have to do is give voice to our wants, but what The IDEA, the 'philosophy of being' discussed in this book, has sought throughout to illustrate is that there has to be a relationship and a congruence (or alignment) between thoughts and emotions or feelings, which are flavoured by our beliefs and attitudes. As well as being part of an external ecological whole, we also comprise an internal ecology. While who we are today has been conditioned by others' attitudes, feelings, and philosophies, if we wish to change, we now have to break free from our conditioning and learn anew who we authentically are, our place in this creation, and the way forward from here.

An awareness of the unity of life will change our values, and therefore our behaviour. Such an awareness of our interconnected existence is transformational. It will cause us to question many of our existing paradigms and those of society around us.

The important thing to remember is that we don't have to make a 100% change in ourselves to achieve a change in our lives. As the Bible explains it, *'I tell you the truth, if you have faith as small as a mustard seed, you can say to this mountain, "Move from here to there," and it will move.'* [191]

The steps we take will be incremental and will build as our confidence grows; for the universe will respond to our efforts, to our consciousness, to our struggling belief, and to our observation.

We should all celebrate when we manifest into reality what we think and seek, but if you are having a bad hair day, do not play the victim. Stop and think – did you manifest that too? If you live fearfully, then you may well attract what you fear.

The energy is yours to create your world – be amazed at how consistently it will do just that!

The rhythm of life - the tuning fork principle

We live in a vibrating and rhythmic universe where the rhythms of the life of one will affect the rhythm of life of another. This has enormous implications for all of us. We resonate in sympathy with what we surround ourselves with. We know this intellectually and intuitively, yet, in our reading, our viewing and our conversations – do we surround ourselves with joy and laughter or with negativity and complaint?

---

[191] Matthew 11 v23

Two matched tuning forks are mounted on resonance boxes. Hit one, and the other vibrates too. This is the tuning fork principle.

> *The matched (same natural frequency) tuning forks mounted on boxes will couple to each other effectively. In other words, put them near each other and hit one. The other will vibrate as well. This means energy has been efficiently transferred from one to the other, a resonance effect. On the other hand, a tuning fork with a different natural frequency will not vibrate when placed near the vibrating fork. Energy is not transferred efficiently.[192]*

Is this principle true when applied other than to musical instruments?

Consider some of the following examples:

In 1656 a scientist, Christiaan Huygens, who had patented a mechanical clock discovered one day that if he placed two clocks together their pendulums would work in unison. This was the case regardless of how the two clocks were adjusted.

In 1971 a researcher, Martha McClintock, found that women who live and work closely together will often begin to menstruate together. No one really knows why[193], but if you think about the tuning fork principle, then it makes some sense.

Research cardiologists have learned that in tackling heart disease, embryonic stem cells might work and that *in culture, they form nodes*

---

[192] New Zealand Physics Resource Bank Retrieved 3 June 2007 from http://www.vuw.ac.nz/scps-demos/demos/Mechanics/TuningForksandResonance/Tuning-Forks.htm

[193] The mechanisms behind menstrual synchrony are not well understood. Pheromones, social cues, and shared environmental factors have been proposed as potential influences, but none have been conclusively proven.

of pulsing cells, presumably immature heart muscle cells, that beat in unison.[194] This occurs because of the same tuning fork principle.

When two objects have the same resonance, they exchange energy strongly *without having an effect on other surrounding objects*. It is about the latent frequency in all objects. This can be demonstrated scientifically and practically, for instance:

> *If you fill a room with hundreds of identical glasses and you fill each one with a different level of wine, each one will have a different acoustic resonance; each glass would ring with a different tone if knocked with a spoon, for example. Then if I enter the room and start singing really loudly one of the glasses may explode if I hit exactly the right tone.*[195]

Electricity unplugged.

In recent times the most startling demonstration of the fact that when two objects have the same resonance, they exchange energy strongly *without having an effect on other surrounding objects* came in the form of wireless electricity. This concept is so startling that it is counter-intuitive and is still a frontier area of science. In 2007, scientists successfully tested an experimental system to deliver power – not just radio signals, but actual power – to devices without the need for wires. This remarkable setup, reported in the journal Science, made a 60W light bulb glow from a distance of 2m (7ft). WiTricity, as it is called, exploits simple physics and could be adapted to charge other devices, such as laptop computers. The system exploits resonance, that

---

[194] Renovating the heart Retrieved 5 April 2008 from http://www.bioheartinc.com/renovating_the_heart_110304.pdf

[195] BBC News Retrieved 7 June 2007 from http://news.bbc.co.uk/2/hi/

same phenomenon that causes an object to vibrate when energy of a certain frequency is applied.[196]

In 2009, WiTricity was demonstrated with mobile phones and televisions being charged wirelessly.

It uses magnetic resonance to transfer electrical energy over distances without physical contact and can work through various materials like asphalt, wood, and stone.

Today it's found in various applications, including:

- Electric vehicle (EV) charging: pads on the ground wirelessly charge parked EVs.
- Consumer electronics: charging mats for laptops, phones, and other devices.
- Medical implants: powering devices like pacemakers and insulin pumps without surgery.

Because the system depends on resonance or matched frequencies, similar to the way a tuning fork works, the transmitting and receiving coils have to be perfectly matched. Consequently, people can walk around the room and in the path of the resonant current and be unaffected as they are unmatched.

The significance of such developments in science is that they reveal the way the unseen frequencies interplay with the material world; however, we are largely unaware of the frequencies that exist in our environment. We are equally unaware of the resonant factors that bear on our lives as we walk this earth as living aerials – receiving, and broadcasting into the universe.

---

[196] BBC News Retrieved 7 June 2007 from http://news.bbc.co.uk/2/hi/

Just because something exists outside our sensory field it does not mean that it does not exist.

The limitations of our conscious perceptual level are readily evidenced. For example, just because our hearing is limited to sound vibrations in the 20 to 20,000 cycles per second (or 20Hz – 20,000Hz)[197] range, it does not mean that is the totality of noise around us. Other creatures in the animal kingdom have significantly higher audio range. A dog, for instance, has a range of hearing of approximately 40 to 60,000 Hz, whilst the sounds produced by Bottlenose dolphins range between 0.25 to 150 kHz.[198] The significance of this lies in the demonstrable reality that different creatures will hear things we don't, and vice versa. Just because something exists outside our sensory field it does not mean that it does not exist.

Everything in our universe vibrates; after all, it is composed of energy. Light itself vibrates, with each colour of the spectrum having its own frequency or wave length. Earth too has a vibrational frequency. In 1952 Dr. Winfried Otto Schumann, professor of Electrical Engineering at the Technical University, Munich, *detected the resonance of earth by measuring the Extremely Low Frequency (ELF) band of vibrating electromagnetic waves. The lowest frequency at which the resonance takes place is 7.83Hz. Higher resonances occur at 14Hz, then 20, then 26, 33, 39 and finally 45Hz.*[199]

---

[197] Wikipedia Retrieved 4 April 2008 from http://en.wikipedia.org/wiki/Hearing_range

[198] Wikipedia Retrieved 4 April 2008 from http://en.wikipedia.org/wiki/Hearing_range

[199] Brain entrainment and Schumann resonance Retrieved 5 April from http://success-nirvana.blogspot.com/2006/11/brain-entrainment-and-schumann.html

As without, so within

Unsurprisingly then, the human body itself is a symphony of sounds and frequencies. We have previously considered the various frequencies of the brain waves; however, the whole body in its various parts has its own frequencies as well.

While it is the brain waves and their resonance that particularly interest us, consider the beneficial consequences of your body and mind being attuned to their environment. Being attuned is beneficial for our physical health and well-being as it allows us to exist in harmony with our internal and external environments. This permits our lives to be lived out in intelligent cooperation with the universe's deeper order.

Have you noticed how your mood changes when you are watching the ocean, sitting in a green and still forest, or listening to different types of music? What is happening is that, in line with the tuning fork principle, your brain waves frequency responds to that of the environment.

Your brain wave frequency will always respond to the environment but, as we have previously canvassed, there are two environments, the external and the internal environment. Meditation and other exercises will change your internal environment and the rhythm of your brain as much as any external stimuli will. Such exercises enable us to be vastly more creative, aware, responsive, and less reactive. As always, we can be more in control of our being than we think we can be.

If we change the frequency of our brain waves, we change the state of our mind because we then resonate at a different frequency and what we resonate with becomes different. In this way, we can create our own reality.

Energy: The link

'If you want to find the secrets of the universe, think in terms of energy, frequency and vibration.' – Nikola Tesla

We live in a world that remains philosophically scientific rationalist, governed by a belief in a Newtonian material universe. This is a world that would have us believe that *what you see is what you get*. This is a world where the public assertion is that we are governed by our senses; a world where our senses affirm our only certainty, the certainty of our individual existence. This unique certainty was encapsulated by Descartes in the phrase: 'Cognito ergo sum' or 'I think, therefore I am'.

This philosophical perspective, effectively denies the ramifications of recent science, particularly Quantum Physics, which confirms that very little in our universe can be seen. This is because regular matter only accounts for 5% of the universe.[200] The other 95%, comprising dark matter (27%) and dark energy (68%), is a total mystery to the scientific community. As Robert Brett, Managing Editor of LiveScience, put it 'Dark matter and dark energy are two of the most vexing problems in science today.'[201] There is, some agreement amongst scientists that what is called dark matter points to an ethereal or intangible quality of the universe.

It is not surprising that science with all its resources is unable to fathom the mysteries of the universe and that humanity is equally unable to discern the unseen connections of the universe, except through the circumstantial evidence of its effects on our lives (consider gravity.)

---

[200] In this chapter I have spelt the word 'universe with a lower case 'u' where I am talking of the scientifically defined concept, and with an upper case 'U' where I am referring to the broader concept of the 'Universe'.

[201] Science, retrieved 14 July 2008 from http://www.space.com/scienceastronomy/mystery_monday_040712.html

Does this mean that we should act as though these connections, conduits, and energy flows of the unseen do not exist? Surely, if we are to maximise our lives in this temporal world, then we need to learn what we can of them, and then act on that knowledge to better our lives.

We live in an unseen, but scientifically established, creational wash. We are not simply individual rational entities, with autonomous wills and intellects, forging our separate destinies in an atomised, mechanistic world. We are, in fact, part of a continuum of energy in different forms with two aspects.

First, as individuals, our mind is essentially an energy field that arises out of the mass of neurological electrical circuitry giving rise to a composition comprising the conscious and unconscious life of an individual. As individuals, each of us radiates a unique energy signature, as does every other material object.

Second, the Universal Mind (or, in scientific terminology, the Unified Field[202]) is the synergy created by the energy fields of all living entities in the seen and the unseen worlds which includes us as individuals. What Quantum Physics demonstrates is that we are a part of a universe where there is an integration of inter-related, interactive, energy fields. We do not exist in isolation from each other or creation.

---

[202] Unified Field Theory (UFT):

This is a hypothetical theory that would describe all fundamental forces and elementary particles in the universe using a single theoretical framework.- Currently, the universe's forces are understood through separate theories: gravity by general relativity, electromagnetism by quantum electrodynamics, and the strong and weak nuclear forces by the Standard Model.

A UFT would unify these disparate theories, explaining them as different aspects of a single underlying field. This could unlock profound insights into the universe's nature and laws.

Previously, we considered the possibility that we are living aerials into the universe. What Quantum Physics demonstrates is that as living aerials it is about power, the spiritual power (for lack of a better word), that we attract to us.

We have seen that the resonance of our individually unique frequency attracts what we tune into and that we are part of a complex interlinked universe where nothing is as it seems to our five physical senses. This universe is expressive of an intelligence that gives purpose to its design and is also accessible to humanity if we become open and aware.

It is worth repeating here that as human beings we are demonstrably more than our five senses. We live in the three dimensions of body, soul, and spirit; three gradations that exist co-continuously with each other, bridged by our consciousness. It is this very bridge to the universe that carries the potential to unleash great change in us.

However far away we might think we are from living our grandest dreams, we are really much closer than we think. It's just that our reliance upon the rational mind can blind us. We are not years, months, or even days away, we are just a little new thinking away. Such thinking means opening ourselves to all the possibilities of life, even as we push towards our goals.

Napoleon Hill, author of *Think and Grow Rich*, (1937) wrote:

> *'Thoughts which are mixed with any of the feelings of emotions constitute a 'magnetic' force which attracts, from the vibrations of the ether, other similar or related thoughts. A thought thus "magnetized" with emotion may be compared to a seed which, when planted in fertile soil, germinates, grows, and multiplies itself over and over again, until that which was originally one small seed, becomes countless millions of seeds of the same brand.'*

I suggest that some of the greatest visions that have been realised in people's lives weren't dreams at all, but beliefs and standards that simply weren't compromised, despite apparent difficulties, other people's ridicule, or the pressures of daily life.

It is often hard to see what is happening oneself and the reason for this is that we mostly only understand (and usually are only able to know) the end results. *'Life is lived forward and understood backwards.'* [203]

Like the fish in the ocean, goldfish never question their environment, for they do not understand it. We too, like goldfish, can swim in our own circular experience of life around and around and around, unquestioning within our own limited stream of consciousness until we face difficulties, even turmoil and commotion. In the resultant unpredictability we can see the boundaries of our existence shift as the tides of life open our paradigms. Change comes out of challenge.

Why is this so?

The answer in short is that we are the material form of pure energy with an infinite reach. Just as we can only recognise the invisible forms of energy when they transform into some aspect of mass, so too we can only see our effect when we cause that energy to be rechannelled through changing our paradigms and so our lives.

Let's look at how this happens.

---

[203] Søren Kierkegaard

Conductivity and definition

In science and common understanding the universe is permeated, held together, and comprised of two things:

- Mass;
- and energy.

Until Einstein, these two were considered as separate things. With Einstein's Theory of Relativity[204], the interchangeable relationship between the two was theoretically demonstrated. Since his time scientists, using particle accelerators, have proven that mass and energy are interchangeable properties. Mass can be converted into energy, and energy can be converted into mass.

In fact, mass is derived out of energy and the mass so formed remains bathed in electromagnetic energy at an atomic level. Indeed, it emits electromagnetic radiation as a constant. Mass gives definition to energy in our sensate world, but energy itself is undefined. It lacks form and substance. By its very nature, it is a latent potential, waiting for the creational impulse in the universe that will cause it to become mass. The relationship between energy and mass is close, intertwining, and from the perspective of mass it is co-dependent.

Consider this:

'If a 2.2-pound (1 kilogram) gold bar absorbs enough energy to heat it up by 18 degrees Fahrenheit (10 degrees Celsius), the mass of the gold bar would actually increase! Conversely, if the bar radiates heat to cool off by the same amount, its mass will decrease by the same tiny fraction.

---

[204] $E = mc^2$

It is important to note that the total energy of the entire system remains the same; no energy is being created or destroyed. The heat energy is simply changing its form to become mass.' [205]

Energy is largely invisible to the naked eye, but it is the force that makes the universe alive. In energy lies potential. In energy lies initiative. Energy can exist without mass, but the same cannot be said in reverse. The universe arose from energy. Science, Hinduism, Taoism and the Bible agree on this point.

'Together with the positive and negative poles of electric energies as well as the attraction and repulsion poles of magnetic energies, the universe can never come to a standstill. In fact, these forces could never be physically unified as one. They remain always discrete and separate. It's a waste of time trying to unify electricity and magnetism, or forces of Ying and Yang, which would take the life out of the universe.' [206]

Energy's creational impulse is demonstrated, for instance, in the creation of a new star from the energy released by a black hole in space.[207] Energy in this context is a causing force, whilst mass (the new star) is the response to the causing force.

The power of energy may also be captured and channelled through the deliberate activities of mankind. Think of electricity lighting our homes and driving industry. Here mankind is the causing force in

---

[205] How Einstein's E=mc^2 Works: Available at: http://www.livescience. com/45714-how-einstein-s-key-to-the-universe-the-mass-energy-equivalence-for-mula-works-infographic.html

[206] The regenerating Universe retrieved 11 August 2007 from http://www.regener-ating-universe.org/10)_How_is_universe_of_energy_structured.htm

[207] The National Space Society retrieved 11 August 2007 from http://www.space. com/scienceastronomy/mystery_monday_050207.html

changing the environment through the use of energy. Certain forms of energy are also channelled by our thinking.

To illustrate how this happens think of a small stream. As a young child I used to love playing around streams that could be partially dammed or were small enough to be diverted into new channels. I was never quite sure where the water would flow as I began putting rocks and debris in the path of it, but the course of the water always changed as the pile of rocks grew. As the water course changed, it then changed its physical surrounds through flooding and erosion. That is similar to the energy fields of our thoughts which, like the water, are fluid and as the energy field of our thoughts change so too does our life, impacting our surrounding environment which forms the water bank of our existence in this life.

CHAPTER 13

Nature or Nurture? Our Genetic Code (DNA) doesn't Determine our Fate

Beliefs become biology

THE IDEA EMBRACED IN THIS book has several singular scientific themes. It has sought to weave them into a philosophy that can underwrite the tapestry of our lives. The central thesis of this philosophy is that we are all called to be participants in a greater existence than our sensory world suggests, and our existing beliefs generally allow.

> **Our beliefs and other non-genetic factors activate our genes, causing them to behave differently and so change our physiology.**

This chapter considers how our beliefs and other non-genetic factors activate our genes, causing them to behave differently and so change our physiology[208]. What is

---

[208] the way in which a living organism or bodily part functions

remarkable is how such changes can then last for multiple generations for better or worse. The fact is that the genes we inherit from our mothers and our fathers are not our fate!

In respect to the science this book has touched on, we have seen that:

- Quantum Physics is urging us to change our focus from the material realm and, instead, focus on the dimensions of the unseen realm and so consider a probabilistic and not a deterministic dimension to our lives;

- *'The brain and nervous system are dynamic structures boiling with change, rewiring themselves second by second on the basis of both internal and external stimuli.'* [209] Indeed, the brain remains plastic throughout our lives. This, and our ability to control the activity of our brains, provide us with a key to changing our lives by changing our thinking; and

- We live in inter-relationship with all living things. There is no such thing as a singular idea, or desire, in life because everything is joined to everything else. Therefore, while we may want to be singular, life is so interconnected that whatever we do, say, or even think, provides multiple responses in a connected environment.

These facts which support the central thesis of The IDEA are further reinforced when we consider recent genetic science. This has shown that not only are our brains plastic and grow, reshaping and changing themselves across our lifespan, but so too does the genome.[210]

---

[209] Energy Psychology Journal Fighting the Fire: Emotions, Evolution, and the Future of Psychology, retrieved 14 February 2011 from http://energypsychology-journal.org/?p=63

[210] A genome is an organism's complete set of DNA, including all of its genes. Each genome contains all of the information needed to build and maintain that organism.

The study of changes in organisms caused by modification of gene expression, rather than alteration of the genetic code itself, is known as epigenetics. Epigenetics explores how our attitudes, behaviour, lifestyle and choices can influence which genes get turned on or off. Your environment and lifestyle can change your genes! This science further highlights how beliefs become biology.

Epigenetics establishes how genes not only do *not* control behaviour, but beliefs (expressed in our behaviour) and our environment influence the responses in our genes. This occurs without affecting our underlying DNA.

We have, in the way genes work, a virtuous circle of complex events that reinforces itself through a feedback loop, as follows:

The external/internal environment activates and influences the gene – affecting the expression of genes – this places the gene in a new external/ internal environment which activates and influences the gene … and so on.

For example, at a purely physical level, how what we eat changes our risk profile to hereditary disease by activating latent genes, as illustrated:

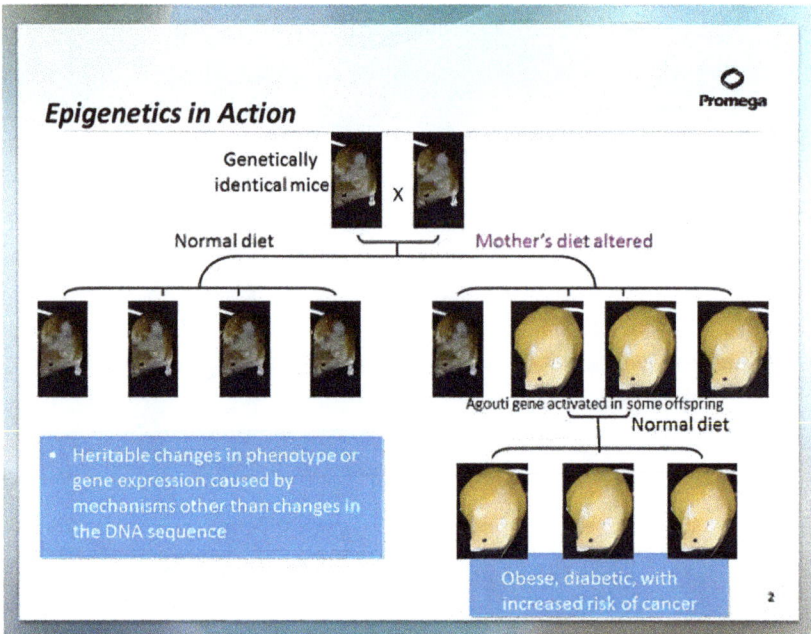

**Figure 13.1: Epigenetics in action – how diet
changes hereditary outcomes211**

This groundbreaking discovery finds its explanation in the science of
Quantum Physics where all matter is recognised as being essentially
composed of energy. As neurosurgeon, Dr. Jack Kruse, wrote:

*'Energy changes the structural and function of matter. Proteins are
a form of matter. Energy sculpts what proteins can and will do and
how they will act in a cell. This is called conditions of existence,
or epigenetics, today.*

*Darwin told you about both. Of the two, he said conditions of
existence were by far more important. Biology has forgotten what*

---

211 Webinar Redux: DNA Methylation Mechanisms and Analysis Methods: September 12, 2012 by Kari Kenefick

234

he said back then, because for 160 years, no one had a clue how epigenetics worked. Now we do.' [212]

Epigenetics is a relatively recent science in which scientists have learned that contrary to established belief, genes can and are turned on and off by signals from our external and internal environments, from outside the cell. Dr. Bruce Lipton, a former medical school professor and cellular research scientist, was one of the first scientists to posit such extra-cellular control.[213] His work has subsequently been validated by other researchers.

But what is a gene and why does epigenetics affect our lives and our world view?

Genes

'Genes have for over half a century easily eclipsed the outside natural world as the primary driving force of evolution in the minds of many evolutionary biologists.' [214]

As the above quote highlights, genes have long been associated in evolutionary science as entities whose characteristics lasted through succeeding generations. So, what is a gene?

A gene may be defined as being:

---

[212] Energy and Epigenetics 6: Quantum Cell Theory, Life as a Collective Phenomena Available at https://www.jackkruse.com/ee-6-quantum-cell-theory-life-collective-phenomena/

[213] Truth about Food and health, 'New Research Reveals That Thoughts Affect Genes', retrieved 11 February 2011 from http://www.thetruthaboutfoodandhealth.com/healtharticles/biology-of-belief-bruce-lipton-genes-cell.html

[214] Eldrige, N. 2004 *Why we do it*, Norton, New York p15

'The fundamental physical and functional unit of heredity; It is an individual element of an organism's genome and determines a trait or characteristic by regulating biochemical structure or metabolic process.' [215]

The genome is the entirety of an organism's hereditary information. Despite early estimates that a human being comprised 200,000 genes, the human genome is now thought to be only composed of between 20,000 and 25,000 genes. A water flea has c. 35,000 genes.[216] More than a third of the water flea's genes are unknown in any other animal and, what is notable for what follows in this chapter, *'those previously unknown genes are due to the nature of the flea's environment.'*[217]

> **It is the environment, not the DNA, that will control the activity of this protein covered group of genes.**

In fact, humans have a similar number of genes to much simpler organisms. With such a clear shortfall in capacity, how does a gene manage? How is it that with a defective gene that leaves an individual susceptible to a cancer, only a very small percentage of people actually succumb?

There are two types of genes. The first type has a regulatory protein cover. This may amount to 50% by weight of a gene and, in the past, this cover was discarded by scientists. The second type does not have the regulatory cover. The second group of genes, which might relate to the colour of our eyes for example, will readily find expression

---

[215] Enotes.com 'encyclopedia of genetic disorders' Retrieved 12 February 2011 from http://www.enotes.com/genetic-disorders-encyclopedia/gene

[216] Brown, M., Wired Science, retrieved 12 February 2011 from http://www.wired.com/wiredscience/2011/02/water-flea-genome/

[217] Brown, M., Wired Science, retrieved 12 February 2011 from http://www.wired.com/wiredscience/2011/02/water-flea-genome/

through the cellular system. The first group, by contrast needs to have the regulatory protein cover removed for the gene to be read by a cell. This happens through environmental signals. These include vibrational signals arising out of the environment, including thought, the frequency of which is aligned to the receptors (refer to the section on the tuning fork principle in Chapter 11). So, it is the environment, not the DNA, that will control the activity of this protein covered group of genes.

The way the gene works is seen as being analogous to the way a computer works. The gene could be described as the hard drive or, as Dr. Lipton put it, the gene *is the organic equivalent of a computer chip, and the cell's equivalent of a brain*. As such, genes store and use information within their design capacity. This, to extend the analogy, includes a range of software programs. The gene effectively extends its apparent capacity in terms of the software program accessed as held on the computer chip.

This means that the input which switches the relevant software program on is as critical as the hard drive or, in this example, the gene itself, in achieving the output. For this reason, until a gene is studied in the context of the energy inputs that it is plugged into, any such study is like trying to explain the design capacity of a computer without plugging it in and studying it through the way it uses software and how those macros [218]in the software work.

If we tried to do that, we would have a very incomplete picture of the real capacity of the computer and its software. For the reality is that the input signals that the gene receives provide the activation of different parts of the gene.

---

[218] a single computer instruction that results in a series of instructions in machine language

Yet this is just how establishment science has sought to study the gene. The result is that such science, together with its limited findings, is also embedded in popular thinking.

Consider this: the newsletter for the students at the Health Science campus of the University of Southern California proclaims, *'Research has shown that 1 in 40 Ashkenazi women have defects in two genes that cause familial breast/ovarian cancer...'* [219]

'Things happen in energy fields before they materialize in the physical domain of our world. Future medicine will be based on controlling energy in the body.'
Prof. William Tiller - Stanford University

So embedded is the deterministic medical view that defective genes cause cancer that most of us will nod wisely in agreement with the statement and expect to see cancer in those women. Yet it is only a partial truth, for the inputs have been isolated from the consideration of the genetic factors. Those inputs are our internal and external environments. There is a slight acknowledgement of this in some circles of evolutionary science, but by and large genes are not seen to be readily adaptive.

Epigenetic mechanisms have been found in a number of studies, *'to be a factor in a variety of diseases including cancer, cardiovascular disease and diabetes. In fact only 5% of cancer and cardiovascular patients can attribute their disease directly to heredity.'* [220] (Willett 2002, Silverman 2004)

---

[219] Church, D., *Genie in your genes*, Elite Books, California ,2007
[220] Lipton, B. *The Biology of Belief,* 2005 Hays House Inc. New York.

Epigenetics has established that the inputs, both the internal and the external environment, are major factors in activating genetic expression and, therefore, of the outcome.

The gene and behaviour

Future medicine will be based on controlling energy in the body (Prof. William Tiller - Stanford University).

To understand the working of genes we have to recognise a first principle that runs like a thread through many chapters in this book and that thread is summarised as, *things happen in energy fields before they materialise in the physical domain of our world.*

Humans occupy an energy field and inhabit a universe made of energy. At an individual level we have seen how the brain operates by sending electrical messages across synapses. We have also seen the way the brain controls all the processes in the body. We have looked at how, every time we feel an emotion or enact a belief, the brain sends chemicals throughout the body that will often give us a physical reaction. Such patterns of behaviour and reaction can become hard wired into the brain.

It is a reasonable extension to recognise that the mental and behavioural release of chemicals not only affects the body as whole, but also parts of the body, including genes. This is exactly what science in the first decade of the twenty-first century has demonstrated.

The well-published author, Dawson Church, summarised this discovery as follows:

'The energy flows in neurons and genes interact with their every process. Memory, learning, stress, and healing are all affected by classes of genes that are turned on or off in temporal cycles that range from one second to many hours. The environment that activates genes includes both the inner environment—the emotional, biochemical, mental, energetic, and spiritual landscape of the individual— and the outer environment. The outer environment includes the social network and ecological systems in which the individual lives. Food, toxins, social rituals, and sexual cues are examples of outer environmental influences that affect gene expression. Researchers estimate that "approximately 90% of all genes are engaged…in cooperation with signals from the environment.'[221]

Science has long held the view that in those instances where the genes in our body have altered in some way, they can cause illness; however, until recently this has been a one-way street of causality. The conviction was: *The gene has caused illness and affected behaviour. Genes held an immutable blueprint for our behaviour, life and well-being.* Epigenetics, however, demonstrates recent findings that it is our beliefs and, therefore, our behaviour, as reflected in life choices, which help shape our physiological reality.

There are many examples of how emotional trauma can affect not simply our psychology, but also our physiology, leading to disease, including cancer. In one example, an ongoing collaboration between the Centres for Disease Control and Prevention and Kaiser Permanente undertook the Adverse Childhood Experiences (ACE) study which considered the relationship between multiple categories of childhood trauma and health and behavioural outcomes later in life.[222] This ten-

---

[221] Church, D., *Genie in your genes*, Elite Books, California ,2007

[222] The Adverse Childhood Experiences (ACE) Study, Retrieved 14 February 2011 from http://www.acestudy.org/

year study of over 17,000 adults found a strong correlation between childhood emotional trauma and adult disease, including that of diabetes, depression, hypertension, heart disease and cancer.

The ACE study has been followed up by the Mitigating Adverse Childhood Experiences (MACE) study. This tracks the correlation between the relief of adult stress (and associated childhood trauma) using Energy Psychology techniques and disease symptoms in adults.

> **Epigenetics demonstrates recent findings that it is our beliefs and therefore our behaviour, as reflected in life choices that will help shape our physiological reality**

The ten-year study established the interactions between emotions and gene expression. The MACE study seeks to demonstrate the possibilities of reversing the damage by switching off that part of the affected gene which has been activated.

Some interventions to support people exposed to ACEs include trauma-informed care, cognitive-behavioural therapy, mindfulness, parenting programs, and social support. These interventions enhance resilience, coping skills, and healing among affected individuals and communities.

While genes may predispose individuals to certain disabilities, there are many diseases and health issues which we know are not caused by either genes or environment in isolation. These include obesity, cancer, diabetes, allergies, heart disease, osteoporosis and longevity. [223]

Epigenetics is opening up as a largely unmapped, new and exciting field in gene-related science, with many large-scale research

---

[223] Nature.com, Largest-ever epigenetic study launched - September 08, 2010 retrieved 14 February 2011 from http://blogs.nature.com/news/thegreatbe-yond/2010/09/largestever_epigenetic_study_1.html

projects being undertaken around the world. In one such project, announced in September 2010, TwinsUK, a research group based at King's College London, and BGI, the Chinese DNA-sequencing powerhouse in Shenzhen, launched the Epitwin Project[224] a study of epigenetic effects in identical twins. This is the largest research project of its kind to date. In launching it the group stated that: *'Researchers hope that epigenetics will help to answer questions about the origins of diseases which we know are not caused by either genes or environment in isolation.'*[225]

The implication of epigenetics is profound. This is because genes, in the neurons of our brain, can be activated by input from our emotive centres is radical and indicates a degree of interconnection and feedback that is at odds with the traditional, linear, cause-and-effect model of genetic causation.[226]

What does this mean for us?

The research into epigenetics demonstrates that in the case of one significant class of genes, our internal environment, as well as our external environment, shapes our biological wellbeing by removing the regulatory protein cover for a gene. To paraphrase Dr. Bruce Lipton, a renowned cell biologist, who has transformed our understanding of the mind-body connection and the role of consciousness in health and healing: It can now be shown that we are not a bundle of chemical reactions at the mercy of our own DNA. While our genes might control biological expression, such as the colour of our eyes, they do not

---

[224] Overall, the Epitwin Project provided valuable evidence for the involvement of epigenetics in complex diseases and underscored its potential as a biomarker for diagnosis, prediction, and personalized medicine.

[225] Ibid

[226] Church, D., *Genie in your genes*, Elite Books, California ,2007

"**By changing your perception, you can change your reality.**"
Dr Bruce Lipton

control biological function. In his study of cells and epigenetics, Dr Lipton found that when he took an active cancer cell from a cancer-affected body, and put it into a healthy medium, the cell behaved normally. His work in the field of epigenetics demonstrates consistently the fact that our internal/external environments, including our beliefs, can change outcomes. Beliefs, literally, become biology.

Our internal environment reflects our emotions, our thinking, and our beliefs. To take control of our internal environment, we must consciously take advantage of the dynamic and ongoing changes that occur in our mind. We need to grow our understanding of what is possible, so that we can now take increasing control over what happens in our lives.

We need to become increasingly self-aware.

Many of our emotions and thought processes occur at an unconscious level and it is only through a process of self-awareness that we can change the effect that these unconscious strata of our minds have on our genes and, more broadly, on our being.

In recent years a new science of neuro-immunology has developed which looks at the relationship between the brain, immune system and emotions and thinking. These processes are not conscious, but can come under conscious control, or can be mediated through thinking and through behaviour. This has led various mainstream practitioners to assert that by changing our

By changing our thinking and our habitual affective responses, we can change our health.

243

thinking and our habitual affective responses, we can change our health.[227]

To achieve change, we need to be body aware. As Dr Daniel Siegel put it, '*much of what happens in the mind is not within consciousness, yet these non-conscious processes have an impact on our health. Bringing these negative thoughts... to awareness is part of basic health, because those thoughts—what in my field are called unintegrated neural processes—are basically like black holes. They have so much gravity to them that they suck the energy out of life. ... They also influence the body itself, including the nervous system and the immune system.*' [228]

By understanding how epigenetics can affect the immune system, we can learn how to improve our physical and mental health. For example, we can find ways to reduce stress and promote positive emotions. We can also adopt a positive outlook on life and focus on our strengths. By making these changes, we can improve our immune system and overall health.

Unfortunately, too often there is a dissonance between our consciously expressed desire or behaviour and the unconscious personal conviction of personal inability or ill health. That unconscious conviction may be shaped or supported by the convictions imprinted on us by culture or other people's beliefs.

Some years ago, I had a total knee replacement due, in part, to a squash injury. Some well-meaning people wanted to tell me all about the pain that was associated with such a procedure. From the outset, I banned any such discussion and worked on a premise of a strong recovery

---

[227] The Unconscious Mind available at http://www.mind-development.eu/unconscious.html
[228] Daniel J. Siegel professor of clinical psychiatry at the UCLA School of Medicine and Executive Director of the Mindsight Institute

with minimal pain. I was up from the hospital bed within hours of the operation (dragging drips and other paraphernalia with me to the toilet) and discharged within three days. The nurses were stunned, and the surgeon was thrilled. Three months later, I was walking through the New Zealand Alps. This is not a unique story, but the point is that I did not allow my unconscious to be fed by the negativity of third parties and, hence, impede my recovery. By extension, our own conviction of a third party's recovery or well-being will help improve or retard their situation.

Beliefs become biology.

CHAPTER 14

Meditation

'People who meditate grow bigger brains than those who don't. Researchers at Harvard, Yale, and the Massachusetts Institute of Technology have found the first evidence that meditation can alter the physical structure of our brains. Brain scans they conducted reveal that experienced meditators boasted increased thickness in parts of the brain that deal with attention and processing sensory input.' [229]

Why meditate?

Why should we seek to meditate, and what has this to do with The IDEA?

Throughout this book we have seen that awareness and self-awareness are central to our beliefs, behaviour and life's outcomes, including well-being.

---

[229] *http://www.physorg.com/news10312.html General Science: January 27, 2006*

When the mind is dominated by dissatisfaction and unawareness it is difficult to feel calm and relaxed – instead we feel fragmented and stressed

Controlling and taming the mind is difficult – it requires training and meditation is a scientifically proven pathway to change.

Because of the loadings of our personal history, culture, and relationships, so much that sits in us as perception is, in fact, simply our creation drawn out of our paradigm of reality; that paradigm assumption will often be based on an outmoded worldview of our body, of matter and of energy as we have outlined earlier.

We can, and do, get caught up in the apparent urgency of everything we must do, seeing it all as important. We can fall into a constant and sometimes scarcely recognised state of perpetual anxiety, tension, and distraction. This is further aggravated by our increasingly 24/7 connectivity with the world around us – a connectivity which, even as it links us to anybody anywhere, increasingly distances us from ourselves and our inner landscape[230].

Meditation can free us from negative thinking and assist us in changing our outlook, which changes our being, which changes our lives. It is not simply a nice way of relaxing, but it is something which, with practice, leads to a permanent and profound change. Meditation does not always involve the emptying of the mind, but it always leads to a replenishing of the mind. It provides an opportunity for our brains to become calmer and our minds sharper as we stop, balance, or investigate the bombardment of external and internal stimuli.

---

[230] Kabat-Zinn, J. Full Catastrophe Living, Bantam Books New York pxl

There are many varieties of meditation techniques and traditions but, in essence, they all seek to help us pay attention to what is happening in the body and mind, in the present moment, without judgement. By seeing more clearly our capacity to regulate emotional reactivity and our cognitive evaluation of unpleasant thoughts, emotions and sensations is strengthened.

This is because it is through a non-judgemental awareness, unhindered by our emotional reactions, that we can assess our paradigms and our beliefs and so open ourselves up to the universe.

- Our mind becomes calmer, and we have clearer thinking.
- We can begin to break the cycles of habitual thinking that dominate our lives.
- Our brain waves slow to Theta, improving our intuition and psychic abilities.
- Meditation creates the space in our being to attract and focus on whatever we choose.
- It allows us to become more aware with the result that we become more responsive and less reactive in our lives.
- As outlined in this chapter – there are also a significant range of researched medical benefits that accrue.

So, we do not need a disaster or a 40-day fast to force our minds to free us from established channels of thinking and so disrupt previously-formed patterns. Meditation provides an alternative pathway.

Types of meditation

There are many forms of meditation. Personally, I favour the wide-angle lens of Mindfulness Meditation. While the practice is Buddhist and lies at the core of Buddhist meditative practices there is no God in Buddhism.

In fact, when asked 'Are you a God?' Buddha is stated to have replied 'No ... I am awake.' It is that 'awakeness' that is the focus of this chapter.

Mindfulness may be seen as the awakening from our self-imposed half sleep of unawareness in which we are so often habitually, but not inevitably, immersed.[231]

Mindfulness Meditation

Mindfulness uses the breath as an anchor. The breath is a constant of which we are aware even as we allow the mind to be open to insights.

Mindfulness meditation, according to Dr. Borysenko[232], '*involves opening the attention to become aware of the continuously passing parade of sensations and feelings, images, thoughts, sounds, smells, and so forth without becoming involved in thinking about them. The person sits quietly and simply witnesses whatever goes through the mind, not reacting or becoming involved with thoughts, memories, worries, or images. This helps to gain a more calm, clear, and non-reactive state of mind. Mindfulness meditation can be likened to a wide-angle lens. Instead of narrowing your sight to a selected field as in concentrative meditation, here you will be aware of the entire field.*'[233]

Mindfulness Meditation expanded.

You may have heard of Mindfulness in connection with 'Vipassana' or Insight Meditation. It is very much about, 'refining our capacity to pay

---

[231] Kabat-Zinn, J. Full Catastrophe Living, Bantam Books New York p473

[232] A pioneer in integrative medicine Dr Borysenko is a world-renowned expert in the mind/body connection. Her work has been foundational in an international health-care revolution that recognizes the role of meaning, and the spiritual dimensions of life, as a part of health and healing.

[233] ibid

attention for sustained and penetrative awareness and emergent insight that is beyond thought but can be articulated through thought.'[234] Such meditation allows us to transcend the problems and pains and sorrows of the moment.

Mindfulness is not necessarily associated with relaxation but is based on a non-attachment whatever the emotional state. It is then possible to find peace and serenity against the odds and in the face of the storms of life.

> **All our feelings, thoughts and sensations are like the weather that passes through, without affecting the nature of the sky itself.**
> (Segal, Williams and Teasdale 2002)

As we become aware of the passing parade of sensations and feelings, images, thoughts, sounds, smells, Mindfulness Meditation shifts us from a conceptual reality to an experiential reality.

Mindfulness may be seen as the awakening from our self-imposed half sleep of unawareness in which we are so often habitually, but not inevitably, immersed.

Awareness, that is being conscious of our internal and external environments, is a central strand that runs throughout the IDEA. Because of its linkage to awareness, this form of meditation is beneficial at many levels. It induces an Alpha or Alpha/Theta brain rhythm even as it opens our consciousness to those spheres of the unseen. I say this without in any sense decrying any other form of meditation and you may prefer another form.

---

[234] Segal, Z.V. et al 2002 *Mindfulness based cognitive therapy for depression* Guildford Press London pviii

It follows then that the key to Mindfulness is not so much what we choose to focus on, but the quality of awareness that we bring to the moment.

So often people will say that they are caught by and entangled by a thousand different thoughts that come into their minds when they meditate and before they know it, they feel as if they are no longer meditating. Does that sound vaguely familiar to you? We get caught up with our reactions to our thoughts; however, while this diminishes our awareness of the present moment, we should recognise that we are still undertaking meditation practice. It is called meditation practice because we never fully achieve it, we simply practice it.

Practicing Mindfulness allows us to move from automatic pilot and letting the mind be as it is. It's not about making the mind empty or still, although that may be cultivated.

As Jon Kabat-Zinn said, 'you can't stop the waves but you can learn to surf.'[235] In other words, in the context of Mindfulness, if you are experiencing thoughts or feeling pain or distress, don't turn away or bury the thoughts. Learn to surf them; be aware of them as you would when watching clouds in the sky.

Mindfulness is about being aware of the passing parade of thoughts and feelings; not trying to hold on to them, not trying to push them away, but simply noticing as you 'surf', accepting, and letting them go.

It is this non-judgemental, non-reactive, quality of awareness that we bring to bear on these thoughts and feelings, as an observer of them, that makes Mindfulness a powerful tool in stress and pain relief and in

---

[235] Thinkexist.com Retrieved 27 April 2008 from http://thinkexist.com/quotation/you_can-t_stop_the_waves-but_you_can_learn_to/252460.html

the treatment of anxiety and depression. In remaining the dispassionate observer, we don't wander down the paths of our incessant, and often habitual, thinking. Instead, the practice of Mindfulness means that we see things as they are, without trying to change them. The constant practice of this is the basis of forming new neural pathways that can in time, lead to permanent change.

'The aim is to dissolve our reactions to disturbing emotions, being careful not to reject the emotion itself. Mindfulness can then change how we relate to and perceive our emotional states.' [236]

Research and meditation.

In recent years, significant research has been undertaken into the effect of meditation on the brain, individual health and wellbeing. As per the quotation at the beginning of this chapter, in one example Dr Sara Lazar[237] at the Massachusetts General Hospital in Boston, USA, and her colleagues found that meditating actually increases the thickness of the cortex in areas involved in paying close attention and sensory processing, such as the prefrontal cortex and the insula [238]. This was the case especially in older people. When this is considered in the context of the chapter on the brain, the implications of such

> **You cannot solve a problem using the same level of consciousness as created it.**

---

[236] Bennett-Goleman, T. 2001 *Emotional Alchemy* Mackays of Chatham plc UK p6

[237] Sara W. Lazar is an instructor in the Department of Psychiatry at Harvard Medical School, as well as a scientist at the Beth Israel Deaconess Medical Center's Mind/Body Medical Institute and an Assistant in Psychiatry in the Department of Psychiatry at Massachusetts General Hospital.

[238] New Scientist 15 November 2005 Retrieved 21 July 2008 from http://www.newscientist.com/article.ns?id=dn8317

increased awareness are strongly in line with The IDEA that we can create our own outcomes through purposeful activity.

In another study on Mindfulness Meditation, it was shown that the results of Mindfulness practices were:

- 87% less heart disease
- 55.4% fewer tumours
- 50.2% less hospitalisation
- 30.6% fewer mental disorders
- 30.4% fewer infectious diseases[239]

In a recent example of research into the power of meditation to 'affect the being', Professor Richard Davidson, a Professor of Psychiatry at the University of Wisconsin-Madison and Director of the Waisman Laboratory for Brain Imaging and Behaviour, spent some time studying the effects of meditation on Buddhist monks and students.

In June 2002 Davidson's associate, Antoine Lutz, positioned 128 electrodes on the head of Mattieu Ricard. Ricard was a French-born monk from the Shechen Monastery in Katmandu, who had undertaken more than of 10,000 hours of meditation.

'Lutz asked Ricard to meditate on unconditional loving-kindness and compassion. He immediately noticed powerful gamma activity – brain waves oscillating at roughly 40 cycles per second – indicating intensely focused thought. Gamma[240] waves are usually

---

[239] The Institute of Public Administration Australia, 'Mapping the futures of generations' Retrieved 3 June 2011 from www.wa.ipaa.org.au/download

[240] Until recently gamma brain waves have received the least attention and research. During moments when bursts of precognition or high-level information processing occur, your brainwaves reach the Gamma state. The Gamma brain wave state corresponds to frequencies of 40Hz or higher.

weak and difficult to see. Those emanating from Ricard were easily visible, even in the raw EEG output. Moreover, oscillations from various parts of the cortex were synchronised — a phenomenon that sometimes occurs in patients under anaesthesia.

The researchers had never seen anything like it. Worried that something might be wrong with their equipment or methods, they brought in more monks, as well as a control group of college students inexperienced in meditation. The monks produced gamma waves that were 30 times as strong as the students'. In addition, larger areas of the meditators' brains were active, particularly in the left prefrontal cortex, the part of the brain responsible for positive emotions.

Davidson realised that the results had important implications for ongoing research into the ability to change brain function through training. In the traditional view, the brain becomes frozen with the onset of adulthood, after which few new connections form. In the past 20 years, though, scientists have discovered that intensive training can make a difference. For instance, the portion of the brain that corresponds to a string musician's fingering hand grows larger than the part that governs the bow hand — even in musicians who start playing as adults. Davidson's work suggested this potential might extend to emotional centres.

But Davidson saw something more. The monks had responded to the request to meditate on compassion by generating remarkable brain waves. Perhaps these signals indicated that the meditators had attained an intensely compassionate state of mind. If so, then maybe compassion could be exercised like a muscle; with the right training, people could bulk up their empathy. And if meditation could enhance the brain's ability to produce "attention and affective processes" — emotions, in the technical language of

Davidson's study - it might also be used to modify maladaptive emotional responses like depression.' [241]

Professor Davidson and his team published their findings in the Proceedings of the National Academy of Sciences in November 2004. The research made 'The Wall Street Journal and Davidson instantly became a celebrity scientist.

Meditating may slow down or prevent the decline in age related cortical structure.

Professor Davidson's study with his students using Mindfulness Meditation also showed that, within a very short space of time, there was a significant change to both their thinking and their immune systems.

In a prior interview on Radio National in 2003, Professor Davidson had this to say about it:

And what we found is that individuals who participated showed a significant increase in activation in left pre-frontal regions of their brain. That was associated with a reduction in the amount of anxiety that they reported. And we also found remarkably that there was a change in the immune system in these individuals, compared to individuals who were in our control group. We found that to be remarkable. Given the brevity of the training, it suggests that meditation was producing systematic changes in both the brain and the body in directions that were positive. [242]

---

[241] Wired Magazine February 2006 Retrieved 22 March 2008 from http://www.wired.com/wired/archive/14.02/dalai.html

[242] Radio National, 'Science meets Buddhism', 14 September 2003, Retrieved 22 March 2008 from http://www.abc.net.au/rn/science/mind/s943369.htm

In a 2011 TED talk on 'How Meditation Can Reshape Our Brains'[243], Dr Sara Lazar, an Associate Researcher in the Psychiatry Department at Massachusetts General Hospital and an Instructor in Psychology at Harvard, noted the following:

> 'As we get older areas of our prefrontal cortex shrink – making it harder to figure things out – what is interesting about the following image is that the 50 year old meditators have the same amount of prefrontal cortex as the 25 year olds suggesting that meditating may slow down or prevent the decline in age related cortical structure.'

This was well illustrated in the image below.

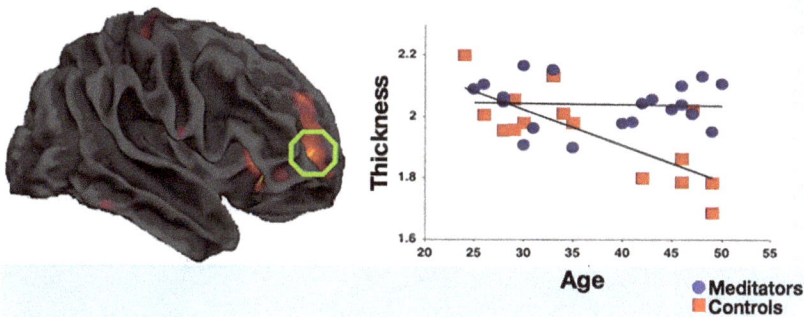

Figure 14.1: Reshaping our brain through meditation[244]

Meditation can literally change our brains and is a genuinely important instrument in reconnecting our inner world of thoughts, feelings, and energy with our outer world of the circumstances we

---

[243] Sara Lazar at TEDxCambridge https://www.youtube.com/watch?v=m8rRzTtP7Tc

[244] https://www.pinterest.com.au/pin/527132331363531682/

attract into our lives. It is the medium through which we can find access to the unseen because of its impact on both our physiology and mental processes.

CHAPTER 15

What holds us back and how to move forward?

It's much easier to tell others what their problems are than to sort out your own. (Mahatma Gandhi)

WHY IS IT SO HARD to understand what is happening, and take effective control of our lives as we live forward? Why is it so hard to grasp and apply the 'possibility thinking' that is the framework of our potential?

There are, in fact, many anchors holding us back in our thinking, based on our own and other people's experiences, fears and thoughts.

We are unaware of these anchors which are a bit like icebergs. The larger and invisible part is buried in our unconscious - that part of our brain that governs habitual thoughts, our emotions and unintentional behaviours. It makes up 90% of our brain.

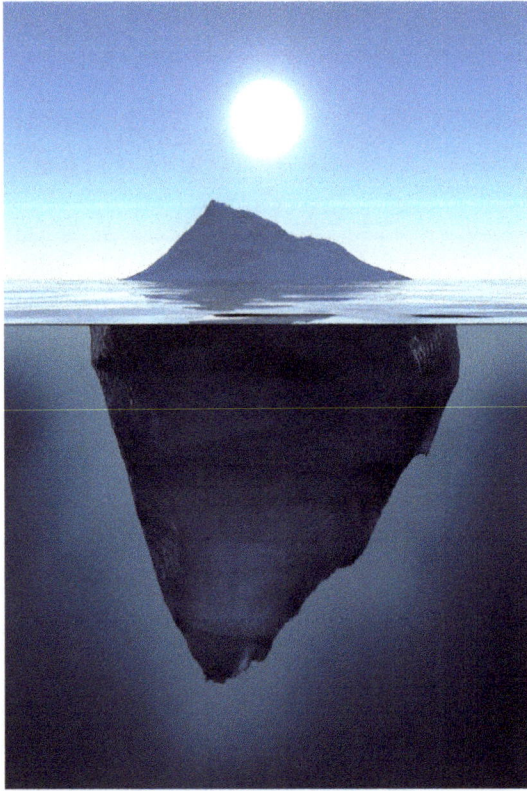

Figure 15.1: The iceberg of our brain[245]

Our conscious mind, the 'visible' part of the iceberg, experiences the results of our unconscious thinking patterns and is left wondering why we just do not seem to be able to lose weight, to be on time, to find our soul mate, get the right job, or to save money.

The prospect of change can be challenging. Often, however dysfunctional our lives are, there is a feeling of certainty about them that is more reassuring than changing to an uncertain future.

---

[245] Image by Patrick Ellis – reproduced with permission

Change can feel unsettling, like losing control over your life. The prospect of navigating a new and unpredictable situation can be anxiety-provoking.

Life is not about the safety of being anchored in the vestiges of some experience. Life is about increase.

There is a 'use it or lose it' aspect to life and its opportunities and if we use our brain, our muscles, our money, or our time wisely, we will experience increase. We need to reprint our brains and make new experiential synapses. It can, however, be frightening to pull up the anchor and sail into the seemingly uncharted waters of new experiences, relationships and opportunities, with all the potential risks they contain.

It takes courage, and it is not always plain sailing – the seas can get rough.

We also need to 'grow our awareness' if we are to make conscious choices and to be in control of our lives. Our conscious awareness has to become our helmsman in life, not the unconscious currents of our being.

Free will is arguably both our greatest gift and also our greatest curse, as it is often shaped by greed, love or fear: Even as we strive to become more conscious, the limbic system can overpower the rational mind at critical moments in our lives.

Safety does not exist in sitting still as the world rushes past us. Nor do we do ourselves any favours by ignoring the possibilities that the universe affords us. Rather, we need to be conscious in using our time, making the effort to be committed to our goals and dreams. That is about using our free will, the pre-frontal cortex.

We have to 'do the stuff' to access the treasure.

The cargo cult mentality

We have to 'do the stuff' because we are on a journey that is real. It is not lazily premised in some artificial ritual in the vague hope that somehow, somewhere, in the fullness of time, something will happen, a bit like a cargo cultist.

You may not have heard about the cargo cult, but it pervades wishful thinking. It all began in Papua New Guinea (PNG) after the Second World War, where a new religious cult started, becoming known as the cargo cult.

The Papuan's highland tribes had been significantly impacted by westernisation and the flow of goods arriving in PNG to support the war effort. These goods were dropped into remote highland villages by way of military aircraft. Numbers of indigenous tribal people simply believed that through certain rituals (such as setting up mock airports) their ancestors would recognise their own and send them these products in the same way that white people seemed to receive them. Thus a characteristic feature of cargo cults is the belief that spiritual agents will at some future time give much valuable cargo and desirable manufactured products to the cult members through following certain rites.[246]

---

[246] Wikipedia Retrieved 12 September 2007 from http://en.wikipedia.org/wiki/ Cargo_cult

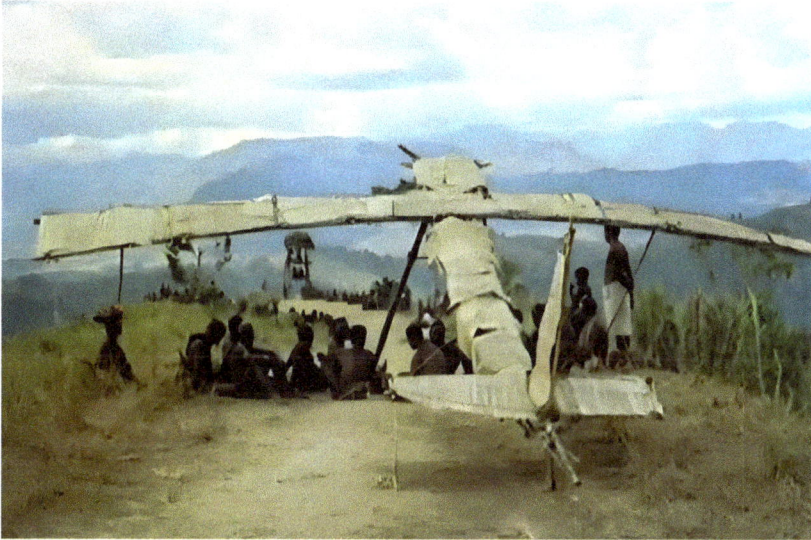

Figure 15.2: Cargo cult mock airport[247]

Problematically, sometimes a military aircraft would actually use the mock landing strip the Papuans had built, and this seemed to affirm the ritual.

They had the wrong cause for an experienced effect.

In our daily lives it is easy to attribute the wrong cause to the experienced effect.

Unlike the cargo cult with its artificial landing strips, what The IDEA proposes is that there is a science that, when combined with a broadly-established life practice, can enable us to unlock the richness of the potential in our lives. To realise our potential, however, we have to do the real stuff, not rest in ritual. The real stuff means working from the inside out to change ourselves and our life experiences.

---

[247] http://www.redstate.com/files/2012/09/Cargo-Cult.jpg

The cosmic triangle

Let's think of our behaviour and progress in life as a triangle. I call this triangle the cosmic triangle as it is characteristic of our personal universe. The cosmic triangle is introduced as a way of representing the past (habitual living), present (new knowledge), and the future (initiative) dynamic of our lives.

Habitual living is, of course, centred in our unconscious being. As was outlined in the chapter on the brain, habitual patterns of behaviour are unconscious forces of habit. By contrast, both new knowledge and initiative can only happen in our consciousness. Our location within the cosmic triangle is determined by our response to these three features.

Habitual living – the first side of the cosmic triangle

'Automatic processes — whether cognitive or affective — are the default mode of brain operation. They whir along all the time, even when we dream, constituting most of the electro chemical activity in the brain.' [248]

The first side of the cosmic triangle is a countervailing force to what the universe would give us, for it reflects our unconscious programming. Habitual living or living without awareness, is formed up in our being and experienced as reactions, patterns of behaviour and assimilated thinking. These have built up over the years of our lives and are often reinforced, not just by our experiences, but also by the culture we live in, together with the media that supposedly informs us. These fixed patterns are the habits that lead to habitual living. We will talk some

---

[248] Casmerer, Lowenstein, and Prelec 2003 9-10

more about this, but for now just remember that habitual living sits in the limbic system, that unconscious part of our being where the limbic system or the 'unthinking centre', influences how we think through the hard-wired circuitry of our brain.

The nature of habitual living

Daily habits establish chemical pathways between the synapses of our brain, modifying its structure and encouraging us to simply stay on the established behavioural track

In talking about habitual living, we are not talking about such natural functions as the heartbeat, or the blinking of our eyes, or breathing, because clearly these are part of the naturally constituted behaviours of our body. We are talking about those imprinted parts of our behaviour over which our conscious control has become mitigated.

This side of the triangle can hold us back from the initiative dynamic. We can find ourselves at the mercy of an outmoded behaviour established in a particular and now irrelevant past circumstance in our lives. As we age and the routines of life establish themselves, this aspect of our habit formation can harden, leading us to become more fixed in our outlook. It requires a real effort on our part to restore plasticity to the brain. It is easier not to think about what we are doing if it seems to be working.

As was outlined, in looking at the plasticity of the brain, our daily habits establish chemical pathways between the synapses of our brain, modifying its structure and encouraging us to simply stay on the established behavioural track.

I should add here that habitual living is also a marvellous thing as we don't have to think about how to drive a car, or how to eat and

If we live habitually we live unaware lives

so on, (once we have learned to do so) every time we get behind a wheel or sit down to dinner. On the downside, habitual living can make change difficult and closes us to what is happening around us. The nature of habitual living is that it is comfortable as it requires little effort and less thought. This is true even when the circumstances around us are mildly discomforting. How often do we put up with things, with people, with situations, because it just requires too much effort to make the change? So, we are running on automatic in many facets of our being.

Have you ever driven to work or home and your mind has wandered and you suddenly think 'how did I get here?' or it's your day off and as you drive you find you are taking the car in a direction towards work without thinking? Your unthinking centre, that part of your being which runs with habits, has taken control of your actions and taken you to work or has otherwise taken charge.

Habitual living affects our relationships and behaviour with our partner. Maybe you have had a row and when you think about it, you can almost call the next action or tactic by the other. Relational disputes can take on the characteristics of a well-rehearsed game, a fact that has not escaped psychologists, not least those who practice transactional analysis.

If we live habitually, we live unaware lives; we live with our unconscious's hands on the steering wheel of our life and, just as happens when we drive habitually, we end up in the same old, same old place.

To the degree we live habitually, to that degree we have surrendered control of our lives.

When these habitual patterns hold us back, they establish the present out of the past as we repeat our behaviour and thinking. Past patterns and experiences can cause us to predict the future from the past. Our habits become a part of our lives as they solve certain kinds of problems and, because they provide a level of certitude, they give us security.

Our experiences also establish what we believe about life and who we are. They form a frame of reference, for example – I know that if I put in so many hours work I will be paid so many dollars. I know that if I eat too much food I will get fat. I might believe that if I do whatever a trusted person (parent, teacher, friend) in my life has told me is important to do then I can be fairly confident of the results. There is an apparent and expected cause and effect which is seemingly proven in many little ways.

There is, however, a problem with habitual living; for if we are relatively comfortable with our life the way it is, then our habitual living will filter out information that is in any way contradictory to our experienced reality. There is no strong intruding external reality forcing us to reappraise our behaviour and beliefs. 'Past programming is a dam holding back the natural free flow of our life stream'.[249] So habitual living blinkers our mind and makes it difficult for us to change. It therefore blocks initiative, which is the third side of the cosmic triangle.

Reducing the impact of habitual living

To change our patterns of behaviour we have to change the lens through which every observation is filtered we need to change our paradigms. We would undertake change because we recognise that the way we

---

[249] Siva, J. & Goldman, B. 1990 *The Silva Mind Control Method of Mental Dynamics* Grafton Books, London.

are thinking may not serve our highest interests. Often this means changing the orientation of thinking. To do this, try to consciously think about the circumstances in which a habit takes over and try to change at least some of them. Drawing on the earlier example, you might regularly vary the route to work or discuss at an opportune moment with your partner the patterns you fall into when there is a disagreement, and so identify an alternative approach.

It is necessary to identify for your mind the positives in making the change. We can picture all the advantages, even as we also list those disadvantages, of changing the old patterns (why not write them down? We can then move to change our thoughts and affirm the positive. In time those positive affirmations will become our reality, our conviction, our new belief. It takes time to re-pattern the neural pathways of the brain and the conscious mind has to work hard to produce more flexible behaviours. This is because the mind is structured in layers, from superficial to profound.

Habitual behaviour resides in our limbic system and our limbic system has a high degree of control over our lives and will either anchor or hold us back. The result is that little changes in our lives. At the superficial level we can scarcely move dust, let alone move mountains. We have to expand our consciousness to retake control of our lives.

As prominent Jungian analyst Dr. James Hallis put it: *'our consciousness is only the ego talking, a fragile wafer cast upon an immense inner sea.'*. The unconscious, as it rises out of that inner sea can cause you to act and think differently to your conscious mind. When it does, you are left asking yourself 'why did I say that?' or 'why did I do that?'

This experience is particularly true when we have chosen to continue our journey in life in denial of our unconscious and its shadow[250] side and imagine that our ego is the totality of our being. In doing this we will lift the shadow to the surface. It will then act like a child, demanding attention at unexpected moments, causing us to behave in ways that are totally out of character. The alternative is to acknowledge our shadow side and get to know ourselves as a precursor to developing our relationships with those around us. In this way, we become more integrated personalities.[251]

So, as a first step in addressing what is holding us back, we have to address the first side of the triangle – habitual living.

In a talk based on his book, *Evolve Your Brain: The Science of Changing Your Mind,* Dr Joe Dispenza describes what I have called the unthinking centre as a partnership between the body and the brain in which the body begins to direct the brain as follows:

'Why is it difficult to change? – Because every time you make a thought you will make a chemical in your body which is released and gives rise to a feeling and this becomes self-reinforcing and gives rise to our state of being. The mind and body work together.

---

[250] The Shadow is the sum of those parts of our being that operate unconsciously on our lives.

[251] Jung, Basel Seminar, 1934: *Love thy neighbors is wonderful, since we then have nothing to do about ourselves; but when it is a question of "love thy neighbour as thyself" we are no longer so sure, for we think it would be egoism to love ourselves. There was no need to preach "love thyself" to people in olden times, because they did so as a matter of course. But how is it nowadays? It would do us good to take this thing somewhat to heart, especially the phrase "as thyself." How can I love my neighbour if I do not love myself? How can we be altruistic if we do not treat ourselves decently? But if we treat ourselves decently, if we love ourselves, we make discoveries, and then we see what we are and what we should love. There is nothing for it but to put our foot into the serpent's mouth. He who cannot love can never transform the serpent, and then nothing is changed*

> **I sometimes wonder whether fabulously rich misers are simply people still locked in a poverty schema in their limbic system; immaterial thinking creating a physical signature.**

The body can influence how we think through these established circuits. Habit is when the body becomes the mind – 'change' is when the mind pulls itself out of the body and puts itself back in the brain. Whilst the body is your mind you can make all the resolutions you want about losing weight or giving up alcohol, but it won't be long before the old habits return and you will be tucking in to whatever you have given up.'

I got to thinking about what Joe was saying, in particular how the body influences the mind. It helped me answer a question that had been troubling me ever since a successful friend committed suicide when he seemed to have it all. In fact, how often do we read or know of people committing suicide and those around that person saying, 'we just don't understand it – he seemed to have everything to live for?'

The answer is that, for some of us, when our body is our mind we are locked into a 'state of being' because our neural networks are so strong that, strange as it may sound, we can feel miserable out of habit. This is so even though our life circumstances say we have everything going our way and there is no need to be miserable anymore. I sometimes wonder whether fabulously rich misers are simply people still locked in a poverty schema in their limbic system; immaterial thinking creating a physical signature. It can happen in so many dimensions of life.

Everything is either growing or dying. If we live our lives in our *un*thinking centre, running on automatic, then our thinking is dulled, our perceptions are limited. We are not allowing ourselves to evolve, but rather we are choosing to stay with addictive habits and emotions. Life still happens but, with habitual living, life can only truly be understood backwards, for we will scarcely be aware of it going forwards.

A developed inner life is indispensable for cognition.

The good news is that you can change habitual thinking, break long-term patterns, and build new neuro-circuits in your brain. Existing knowledge in the right mental frame will then maintain our lives. New knowledge will allow us to grow. We can, therefore, consciously insist on a new state of mind – but to rise above these hard-wired circuitries takes an act of will. If we do not think new thoughts, we are in a grave situation. This is literally so, for we become buried in our own mental detritus.

In summary, habitual living is part of the problem because, as we have seen, we get into habits, into patterns of behaviour which become unconscious or unthinking. We need to be much more aware, more conscious, of what is driving us. To change our lives, we have to create a more effective dialogue between the conscious and the unconscious. We also need to change the hard wiring of our brain built up through the programming of repetitious behaviour which leads to habitual living.

Remember: *Nerve cells that fire together wire together.*

New knowledge acquired – the second side of the cosmic triangle

Importantly, there are two other sides to the cosmic triangle. The second side is *new knowledge acquired* which will then lead us to the third side as we then act on it - we take the *initiative*. Initiative and new knowledge go into partnership. This partnership takes us past habitual living. But what is the nature of knowledge? What we understand by the nature of knowledge will shape our response to it.

There have been several philosophical approaches over the centuries to the theory of knowledge, otherwise known as epistemology. As noted earlier in this book, in recent centuries knowledge has been understood in the Western mind as being dualistic in nature. The knowing of a human is separate from our knowing of nature, creating two streams of knowing; with the human mind simply projecting its thoughts into nature out of its observations.

Knowledge from this perspective can feel quite cold and sits like an inert chemical on the landscape of human cognition because, in this instance, humanity is seen as examining the reality of nature in some detached, objective fashion.

More recently though, as we found in considering Quantum Physics, the prevailing philosophical-scientific view is that we live in a participatory universe where, 'our minds are essentially an organ of the worlds own process of self-revelation ... Nature's reality comes into being through the very act of cognition.' [252]

In terms of Quantum Physics, this means that there is no phenomenon until it is recorded and recording a phenomenon can play tricks with its reality. For example, remember the question of whether light is seen as a wave or a particle and how the observer changes the phenomenon?

While science doesn't confirm minds create reality, it highlights the crucial role our minds play in shaping our experience of the world.

---

[252] Tarnas, R.1993 *The Passion of the Western Mind,* Ballantine Books, New York. p435

Thus, knowledge in a participatory universe is an act of co-creation between human cognition and nature, between the observer and the observed.

This is quite a staggering concept. What it means is that '*a developed inner life is therefore indispensable for cognition, as the imagination directly contacts the creative process within nature, [and] realises the process in itself and brings nature's reality to conscious perception.*'[253]

So, because we do not know what we do not know, new knowledge is the key to both our creative growth and our long-term survival. This new knowledge supports initiative, the third side of the triangle, and allows us to move forward. We must, therefore, use the new knowledge.

Initiative – the third side of the cosmic triangle

Many people have a desire to effect change in their lives and we call this desire initiative. This is the third side of the triangle. Initiative is a product of our will and new knowledge. It is the opposite of inertia. Initiative, as we have seen, sits in the pre-frontal cortex of our brain. Our will, when combined with new knowledge, causes us to rise above our circumstances and then to think and act differently despite how we may be feeling.

The formula is simple:

New knowledge plus initiative overcomes habitual living.

---

[253] Tarnas, R.1993 *The Passion of the Western Mind*, Ballantine Books, New York. P435

In this life nothing stays still. If we settle for the status quo in our lives, we become subject to the ravages of the Law of Entropy,[254] where stagnation sets in and disorder arises as our brains plasticity hardens. The Law of Entropy applies to us as it does to all of creation. Basically, it suggests that things that are unattended run down. Try leaving a tidy house and returning to it after a year and you will see deterioration. Relationships break apart if we don't attend to them, and gardens become unkempt.

Use it or lose it. This is the Law of Entropy.

New knowledge not acted on wastes away and is dissipated, like unused muscles. Unapplied, we forget what it was we had learned.

This should not come as a surprise. Many of us have been on training courses and have discovered that if the course is not followed up by application, then there is a rapid loss of knowledge.

So it is in all dimensions of life. Nothing remains the same, everything either de-generates or it re-generates. We must act on newly acquired knowledge! More than that, unless we do respond to the new knowledge we have acquired, we may even lose what we have gained on our life journey to date.

The creative power of knowledge in this participatory universe makes it the key to our personal development and growth through its subsequent enactment in our lives. In our taking the initiative.

Personal development is hard work. It takes conviction, time, focus and application. Most people don't change their personal reality in

---

[254] Simply put this second law of thermodynamics says that energy of all kinds in our material world disperses or spreads out if it is not hindered from doing so. A hot pan cools; cells die and so on.

any consistent way because they are not focussed enough on what they have learned to meaningfully apply it; nor do they really believe that they have the power to significantly change their personal world, despite being given the information. Without such conviction, or belief, we will not consistently apply new knowledge.

If we are to change our personal world it will require both focus and maintained effort. It takes focus to keep our prefrontal cortex involved. Remember, this is where the seat of our will resides.

> **'When our evolutionary predecessors gathered on the African Savannah millions of years ago and the leaves next to them moved, the ones who didn't look are not our ancestors.'**
> (Al Gore)

Persistence in maintaining focus is often the presenting problem to changing our lives and our situation. Even if we momentarily believe that we attract those things that we focus on, how long do we maintain focus? How long do we remain aware; how long before we become distracted by the next new idea?

Failure to develop awareness may prove personally costly. As Al Gore[255] points out – 'when our evolutionary predecessors gathered on the African Savannah millions of years ago and the leaves next to them moved, the ones who didn't look are not our ancestors.' [256]

Our attention, however briefly, should be drawn to any hints of change in our surroundings. It was a survival mechanism back then and it remains important today. It is all about awareness.

---

[255] Al Gore (born March 31, 1948) is an American environmental activist, author, business person and former journalist. He served as the forty-fifth Vice President of the United States from 1993 to 2001 under President Bill Clinton.

[256] Gore, A. 2007 *The Assault on Reason* Bloomsbury Publishing Plc London

Rather than being eaten by unseen 'predators' in our daily lives, we need to focus on the changes and possibilities in both our external and internal environment.

We have a responsibility to:

- acquire new knowledge;
- take the initiative; and
- act upon it consistently.

We cannot afford to have closed paradigms if we are to succeed beyond our present dreams.

Like it or not, life is a perpetual classroom.

CHAPTER 16

Conclusion –
Tear the walls down

'Faith plus focus plus follow through equals achievement, and many people fail because they just don't have the faith in themselves, while others have the faith in themselves, but they don't focus.' [257]

A S WE ARRIVE AT THE conclusion of this book, it is time to tear down the walls of our paradigms and look beyond ourselves. We have seen that there is more to our lives than the senses alone can reveal. We have been on a journey in this book, a journey that has sought to expand our thinking into the realms of the possible and the probable, underpinned by a clear philosophical paradigm which I have called 'The IDEA'.

This has been a journey revealing how current science forces us to reappraise how we should look at our existence.

---

[257] Let us reason Retrieved May 27 2007 from http://www.letusreason.org/Pop-tea1.htm

We started with a recognition that our thoughts penetrate the interstices of the universe and make tangible the intangible foci of our lives, as we form up our thoughts, charging them with emotion. Remember that things happen in the energy field before they materialise in the physical world. Not least is this true at the physiological level. Remember too that recent findings in the field of Epigenetics demonstrate that it is our beliefs and, therefore, our behaviour, as reflected in life choices, which help shape our physiological reality.

Throughout this book we have seen that awareness and self-awareness are central to our beliefs, behaviour and life's outcomes, including well-being. This means both recognising and understanding our own thoughts, emotions, and motivations.

This book is only intended as a taster of many topics; the rest is up to you as you shoulder your backpack, or swag as we call it in Australia, and continue down the road of life.

On the journey, as you discover the deeper truths of this life and live it as God intended it to be lived, drawing what you need into your life, others will find you. As the founder of Taoism, Lao Tzu said, back in 500 BC:

'Passing by on the road they will be drawn to your door. [because] the way that cannot be heard will be etched in your voice. The way that cannot be seen, will be reflected in your eyes.' [258]

In other words: the power of inner transformation attracts others. It suggests that when you live authentically and embrace deeper truths, you radiate a certain energy that will draw people to you.

---

[258] Lao-tzu: Tao-te Ching Retrieved 17 July 2008 from http://cindylellis.wordpress.com/words-to-live-by/real-magic-wayne-dyer/

The journey that we are called on to travel is one that is deeply unsettling at many levels. This is because it demands that we continually re-evaluate what we are doing, how we are responding, and what our behaviour is.

- It is a journey that demands old mind-sets be broken.
- It is a journey that will take us into uncharted waters of personal experience. It may even take us into the realms of chaos when we first embark on it.

The old saying is that through crisis comes change, because sudden change or crisis can force us to examine old friendships and old habits. For many this is simply too unsettling, and they will turn around and abandon the quest to deeper living – leaving the question: 'What will you do?'

At the end of the day the distance between having it all, and not, is usually only as great as you think it is, and to cover the distance all it takes is the first step, for, as the Chinese philosopher Lao Tzu also said:

The journey of a thousand miles begins with a single step.

Acknowledgements

Writing this book has been a rewarding journey, and I'm grateful for the incredible support I received along the way.

This book wouldn't be what it is today without the unwavering support of my wife, Grace. Her patience as I revised countless drafts and her keen eye for detail were invaluable throughout the writing process. Special thanks are due to Jane Greenslade, whose expertise helped me craft a compelling introduction, and Dedré van Tonder, whose tireless editing after hours ensured the manuscript was in top shape for submission.

To all of these generous people I would like to express my most deep feelings of gratitude for their support, insight and encouragement.

Notes

_____

_____

_____

_____

_____

_____

_____

_____

_____

_____

_____

_____

_____

_____

NOTES

_____

_____

_____

_____

_____

_____

_____

_____

_____

_____

_____

_____

_____

_____

_____

_____

www.ingramcontent.com/pod-product-compliance
Lightning Source LLC
Chambersburg PA
CBHW052015030426
42335CB00026B/3157